The Evolution of a Psychiatrist *Memoirs of a Woman Doctor*

Beulah Parker, M.D.

The Evolution of a Psychiatrist

Memoirs of a Woman Doctor

Yale University Press
New Haven and London

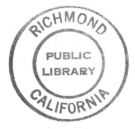

Published with assistance from the Louis Stern Memorial Fund.
Copyright © 1987 by Yale University.
All rights reserved.
This book may not be reproduced, in whole
or in part, in any form (beyond that
copying permitted by Sections 107 and 108
of the U.S. Copyright Law and except by
reviewers for the public press), without
written permission from the publishers.

Designed by Sally Harris
and set in Garamond type by Rainsford Type.
Printed in the United States of America by
Halliday Lithograph Corporation, West Hanover, Massachusetts.

Library of Congress Cataloging-in-Publication Data

Parker, Beulah, 1912–
    The evolution of a psychiatrist.

    1. Parker, Beulah, 1912–   . 2. Psychiatrists—
United States—Biography. 3. Women psychiatrists—
United States—Biography. 4. Women psychoanalysts—
United States—Biography. I. Title. [DNLM:
1. Physicians, Women—personal narratives.
2. Psychiatry—personal narratives. 3. Psychoanalysis—
personal narratives. WZ 100 P238]
RC339.52.P374A3 1987   616.89'0092'4 [B]   86–28069
ISBN 0–300–03371–0

The paper in this book meets the guidelines for
permanence and durability of the Committee on
Production Guidelines for Book Longevity
of the Council on Library Resources.

10 9 8 7 6 5 4 3 2 1

To Otto
who insisted that I tell my story

Contents

Preface

 This is the story of a troubled girl from a troubled family who, by slow and painful steps, became a woman, a doctor, a psychiatrist and a psychoanalyst. She began life three-quarters of a century ago, and grew up within a small segment of upper-middle-class American society—a subculture whose customs and mores were as different from other American subcultures as were those of the Zulus.

Her early world no longer exists anywhere.

In this book I present an account of her life, in the hope of illustrating graphically the kinds of relationships and experiences that promoted her personal and professional growth, using incidents that exemplify significant conflicts at each developmental stage. I demonstrate the way coping mechanisms and characterological attitudes were gradually modified by changing circumstances, enabling her to break away from a non-intellectual, conservative, psychologically disturbed family environment to enter an intellectual "man's profession" almost unheard of among the people she knew throughout her early years.

The story is my own.

The best way to make a point is to present concrete illustrative material which others can evaluate for themselves. I hope that this story will be of interest to members of the mental health professions as a longitudinal study in personality development, but I also hope that young women aspiring to enter any of the professions under very different cultural conditions will find it of at least historical interest, and that they will be able to identify with much in the experience of this woman from another era even while living in the modern world of "equal opportunity."

This account is not a self-analysis, although I do try to indicate how early experiences influenced later life behavior and attitudes toward my professional work. It is a subjective account of experiences that seemed crucial in developing the qualities of heart and mind required to deal therapeutically with the deeper levels of human motivation. In presenting it, I hope to dispel stereotypes about psychiatrists and psychoanalysts and to show that more than one personality type may be successful in these professions.

Throughout this book, I speak of my family members only to indicate how my feelings about them affected my own development. Their story has already been told in *A Mingled Yarn* (Yale University Press, 1972), where, as many have already guessed, I disguised my alter ego as Amy Carpenter, the mysterious informant to Dr. Parker, and attempted to convey the family climate in which my brother developed before becoming overtly schizophrenic in later life. The purpose of that book was to evaluate the role that modes of family interaction and ways of thinking played in creating his disturbance. In this book, I hope to show that not only early influences but the totality of life experience and relationships with people determine personality growth and development.

In the second half of the book, I discuss those aspects of nearly forty years in private practice that may be of interest to non-professional readers as well as to members of the mental health professions.

Background

For the benefit of those who have not read *A Mingled Yarn,* I shall briefly sketch my family background history and the major events that affected the family during my early life, all of which is relevant to my own development.

To a certain point in its history, my family exemplified fulfillment of the American Dream. Ancestors in the direct line fought as officers in the American Revolution and a few in the Civil War. Genealogical records reveal that in those eight early American generations both the men and the women were successfully functioning solid citizens—some quite colorful and a few quite eccentric, but all worthy of respect in our eyes.

I was brought up to take pride in my family background and in the fact that I was eligible to join the Daughters of the American Revolution. I occasionally even thought of doing so until Mrs. Roosevelt's resignation, precipitated by that organization's refusal to let Marian Anderson sing in Constitution Hall, made me realize the insensitivity and intolerance bred by overvaluing the length of recordable lineage. (By that time in my life, Mrs. Roosevelt had become an important role model for many women of my generation, and had caused me to question many of my own values.)

At that time also, I first began to take a serious look at what had gone on in the lives of those members of the older generations of my own family whom I knew. Only as an adult could I allow myself to ask questions that might explode "family myths" passed along by my parents and seek the truth about the lives of my grandparents from more remote relatives who could be more objective than my parents could be.

It was in my grandparents' generation that the American Dream began to become a nightmare. I had to know quite a bit about psychiatry before recognizing that fact. It required experience with patients to teach me that character traits which make for great success in big business are quite opposite from those that make good husbands and fathers, and that when there is too great a discrepancy between the personalities and value systems of husband and wife, tension can be set up within a family that has a deleterious effect upon the children. It eventually began to dawn on me that my grandfathers and grandmothers were totally different kinds of people despite the long years spent locked in "Holy Matrimony," and that these personality differences had something to do with the sad outcomes to the lives of most of their children.

My maternal grandfather was brought up in the family of a prosperous businessman in a small Ohio town. He came to California to work for the newly founded Southern Pacific Railroad and eventually became one of its vice-presidents. Early on, he met and married the winsome and pampered late-life child of an elderly widow from Wisconsin who had brought her daughter to California to seek better opportunities for a suitable marriage. I had always been told that theirs was the love match of the century, but much later in my life learned that in many ways their marriage had been a disaster that was never openly acknowledged. Grandmother went through a period of hysterical blindness following discovery that her husband had been having an affair with another woman, but eventually cured herself by Christian science and ended up as a bland, sweet little old lady. After retiring from the railroad, Grandfather devoted his life to reading the Bible. All day, every day. Five of their six children either died tragically young or were trapped in miserable marriages.

My paternal grandfather was the son of a successful architect who had migrated from New England to New Orleans. At the age of thirteen, he enlisted as a messenger boy in the Confederate Army, was wounded in the lung, and later developed tuberculosis. Traveling across the Southern states to seek a better climate, he met and married a fiery, ambitious Missouri mountain girl from a fanatically fundamentalist family. They settled in rural California near San Francisco in what is now fashionable Marin County. He, an inventive but ineffectual dreamer, worked only intermittently. His four children, although raised on tales of past family glory, lived in relative poverty until the eldest, my father, took over most of their support at the age of nine by selling newspapers in San Francisco.

Everyone agrees that my father was one of the most handsome, brilliant and promising young men who ever lived. While still a teenager he had organized groups of newsboys into a profitable distribution business, put himself through one year at the University of California, and, in spite of his family's poverty, was invited to join one of the most desirable fraternities. Then, rapidly working himself up in the newspaper world, he became the right-hand man, first to William Randolph Hearst, Sr., and then to Medill McCormick, who owned the *Chicago Tribune* until his death. When the paper was taken over by McCormick's brother Robert, my father somehow managed to incur his enmity and left journalism to start a business of his own. From then on, everything went down hill.

I have never known the truth about my father's various business ventures because I tried with all my might to separate myself completely from anything connected with them. All I knew for most of my life was that when setting up his businesses, my father tended to involve my mother in the corporate structure, knowing that she would sign anything he put before her. This was legal, but to the minds of his children it was questionably ethical since my mother knew nothing whatsoever about business. I also knew that he felt the *Tribune* had persecuted him with adverse publicity and wrecked every business he tried to set up. Eventually he sued the paper for libel.

Most of the rest of his life, and the life of our family, was consumed in the battle against this mighty adversary with all its various political connections. After many years, the suit finally came to trial. My father lost, as everyone had predicted from the start. In his old age he then went about trying to found a church and I'm sure that if he were alive today he would be giving Jerry Falwell some stiff competition.

A young man of this temperament met the naive, petted daughter of the mighty railroad vice-president at a fraternity dance—met a young girl who had been brought up in a fashionable world of social and financial security, full of idealism and romantic notions. After a two-year engagement during which he was working in another city and to all appearances more or less forgot about her until questioned by her father about his intentions, he finally managed to take time out from his preoccupation with business to marry her. From then on, as long as he could, he gave her and their children every advantage and material possession their hearts could desire but paid attention to them only intermittently.

Beginning when I was twelve, and for the next twenty-five years, my mother and father lived in different cities and saw each other only three or four times although my mother wrote him long letters about his children almost every week. His replies consisted of three or four lines every six months or so, usually saying that he was about to wind up his affairs and would be arriving a week from Thursday. Mother was always prepared for his arrival, insisting that he would show up at any moment. A telegram would then arrive, postponing the visit until three weeks from Friday. This game went on for twenty-five years.

Each time my mother insisted that he would surely arrive to continue their blissful marriage as he had promised, and that any child who didn't believe it was disloyal to a loving father whose only thought was for the welfare of his children. One day, after twenty-five years, he showed up exactly when he had said he would, as casually as if he had been away for the weekend. They spent their last fifteen years together happily, dying within six months of each other in their mid-eighties.

There is no evidence that in all the years of separation my father was involved with any other woman. He said that he wasn't, and everyone believed him, including my sister, to whom he was the devil incarnate.

We all believed, and I believe to this day that he was just too obsessed with his battles to think about anything else.

Feelings about all that had much to do with creating ambivalent self-images in the three mixed up children of that marriage.

My nine-year-older sister was, from earliest childhood, charming, witty, and well-liked by almost everyone. She was also totally egocentric, unrealistic, and subject to numerous forms of psychosomatic disease which made her a semi-invalid a good deal of the time. Throughout her lifetime she was obsessed by a consuming hatred for her father and anxiety over the fate of her mother. Deserted at the age of eighteen by her childhood sweetheart, she married the next man who asked her, had two children, and was divorced when the youngest was eight. Not long after that, she re-met and rapidly married the man who had deserted her—the first and only love of her life who by then had acquired four children and was also divorced from a psychotic wife. For thirty years they lived together in utter chaos, both refusing to face the fact that her husband was not a genius who would soon be rich and famous— a "folie à deux" not unlike that in which her parents were living. Chronic alcoholism killed her.

My four-and-a-half-year-older brother, his spirit crushed from earliest childhood by the impact of a well-meaning but overwhelmingly dominant and autocratic father, became a frustrated artist. Caught in a conflict between what he was and what he felt he was supposed to be, he gradually became a megalomanic schizophrenic with delusions of being the Messiah, and committed suicide in his early forties.

Research studies on the families of people who become schizophrenic have found that in many cases, the relatively "well" child enters one of the mental health professions. I was that child, who ended up in psychiatry and psychoanalysis. This story is an attempt to show the people and experiences which helped me to avert the kinds of disaster that befell my siblings.

The Evolution of a Psychiatrist   *Memoirs of a Woman Doctor*

1 How But
Not Why

From the age of seventeen, when I first entered college, I was essentially on my own: my parents gave me complete freedom to make my own choices and to rally from mistakes in my own way. Parents can give no greater gift to a young adult, regardless of their own motivations for allowing such freedom.

My mother had her own ideas of what would constitute a "good life" for her daughter—ideas that varied greatly from mine. But she gave moral support to whatever I undertook, no matter how strange it seemed to her, and never wavered from that position. My father, although not a direct part of my life past childhood, was a potent force in the background through his influence on my mother, and at the time his lack of interference with my life meant to me that he tacitly approved of what I was doing, or at least of me as a person. This was important to me, even during the years when I thought I hated him.

I probably couldn't have tolerated all the ups and downs in my life without the belief that I had my parents' respect and approval. Both of them, I think, did give me their approval when they thought about me at all, but I didn't realize for many years how seldom that was.

So I became a "liberated woman" in an era before there was such a term—liberated by the attitude of my parents, liberated by necessity from the world in which I had grown up, and later liberated by the entry of the United States into World War II, which gave professional women opportunities they had never had before. Eventually, the greatest liberation of all was made possible through psychoanalysis, which removed crippling emotional burdens from the past and enabled me to make use of those opportunities in true freedom.

I had grown up in a conservative segment of upper-middle-class society, where women were expected to go to college but few had any inclination to enter professions such as law or medicine, let alone psychiatry or anything connected with emotional disturbance. Regardless of all that liberation, it was astonishing to me, and to everyone who knew me, that I decided to become a psychoanalyst. Very few people in the world I came from ever heard of such a thing in the 1920s and 1930s, and the ones who had tended to ridicule it, as many people still do today.

Psychoanalysis never was a prestigious profession except within a small group of other professional people. Dark places in the human mind are frightening to the average person, even a well-educated one, and those who occupy themselves with what goes on there are apt to be considered slightly crazy or given to possessing occult power. One time in the 1950s, I was visiting a dude ranch in New Mexico—a friendly place where a group of charming, cultured women usually gathered for coffee before starting out on a day's ride. We had all gotten along splendidly for several days until, quite inadvertently, I let it slip out that I was a psychiatrist. The whole group immediately froze into a state of polite withdrawal. One of them later came up to me in awe saying, "I always *knew* there was something special about you. It was your burning eyes! They see right into my soul!" Although I managed to convince her that I didn't read minds while on vacation, things were never quite the same between me and the others. That kind of thing has happened to me more than once, and probably will again.

From my earliest days, something drew me toward an interest in psychoanalysis, whether I knew it or not. In retrospect, I think it was almost inevitable that I would enter some such field. However, to become a psychiatrist, one must first become a doctor, and for a woman of my background becoming a doctor was almost as unheard of as for anyone, male *or* female, to become a psychoanalyst. I had always attended schools and a college specifically dedicated to the idea of educational equality between men and women, and my women classmates and I were given the opportunity to follow any line of study we chose. But for a girl from my particular segment of the cultural group that attended those schools to *choose* to be a doctor or a lawyer was pretty rare. We were educated as well as our brothers and were expected to use our brains as well as our bodies to achieve success in life, but we were expected to use them in occupations suitable for *women*. Today things are very different for young women from similar schools, but that's the way it was back then.*

If college women of my day planned to enter a profession, it was more or less assumed that it would be at some level of teaching, including college teaching, or writing or something in the art world, if we had the talent and interest. It was not absolutely assumed that we would marry, but it *was* assumed that if we did we would marry men of status, have families, and help in the education of our children. We were expected to be the intellectual equals of our husbands, to take an intelligent interest in politics, and to understand their work and its importance in their lives. We were expected to sit on the boards of charitable organizations, organize fund-raising drives, and take part in the women's auxiliaries of hospitals. We were supposed to *complement* the work of professional men, not to compete with them. The few who did, and indeed there were a few, were apt to be considered oddballs

---

* It might be of interest to illustrate the point with a few statistics. From Bryn Mawr, which has always been among the colleges foremost in promoting "feminist" ideals, under 3 percent of 5,349 graduates between the years 1900 and 1945 became either doctors or lawyers, in spite of the fact that the college prided itself on outstanding courses in all the laboratory sciences and offered a premed major. I was one of three out of a class of 122 students in 1933 who became doctors, and we had no lawyers. During the next two decades, the percentage increased to just over 6 percent, and in the following two decades doubled again, to 14.2 percent. In view of the pressure on educated women to enter professions today, I expect it will go higher in the years to come, although it is interesting to see that although doctors outnumbered lawyers up to 1965, the number of lawyers has surpassed them in the twenty years since.

by their peers, and nobody, least of all myself, wanted to be thought of as one of those. I was far too anxious to be accepted by those who "fit in."

Even if I had contemplated entering a "man's profession," the very last kind of work for which I would have considered myself qualified was that of a doctor. Ask almost anyone in the fiftieth reunion class at Bryn Mawr. Among them all I was undoubtedly the least likely candidate for a medical career. When those women knew me, I couldn't even remove a splinter from someone's finger, including my own. I was prone to faint at the sight of blood, gag at the very mention of pus, and turn pale if I caught the slightest whiff of antiseptic in the fluids that were used to clean our halls. Never at any time in the first twenty years of my life had I ever expressed or even secretly harbored the slightest desire to be a doctor, nurse, or any other kind of person connected with hospitals or illness.

As for personal contact with the medical world, I had had none and didn't want any. In fact, my only goal for my future life was to be a successful wife and mother, and I think I was the only one in my class to say so on a questionnaire designed to elicit future career interests from seniors. Even the idea that I might marry a doctor seemed pretty far out in my family. My mother was a Christian Scientist, and my father was as firm in his attitudes about doctors as he was about everything else. To him doctors were, for the most part, charlatans who exploited the gullibility of their innocent victims. If I had insisted on falling in love with a member of this questionable breed, he might magnanimously have granted that the one I had chosen was an exception to the rule. He might have tolerated having a doctor in the family but would never have encouraged it. He had never been ill a day in his life and didn't expect anyone else to have any ailment that couldn't be cured by will power.

Although Mother was a practical Christian Scientist when expedient, recognizing that someone with specialized training might occasionally be required to carry out some mechanical tasks related to the body, she saw little need for medical intervention except to set a bone, stitch up a gaping wound, or deliver a baby. Fortunately her offspring were by and large very healthy, and the few doctors called upon to stitch or set were transients who came briefly. No kindly old family physician lurked in the wings to capture my love or admiration, and as a matter of fact my one contact with a doctor in early childhood left me with my own rather dour view of the healing profession.

At the age of five my chin, raked by an iceskate in a game of "crack the whip," needed stitches. The poor doctor called upon to render that service had bad luck. He underestimated both my mental age and the degree of rage that can be generated in a child who feels humiliated by condescension. When he laughingly tied a bandage on the top of my head to make me look like "a bunny rabbit with big ears," I looked him straight in the eye and bit his finger to the bone. Why he didn't sue my family I don't know, except that people were not quite so ready to sue in those days. I do know that he was the last doctor I would allow to come near me for years. Mother reminded me of this when I decided to become a doctor myself.

So much for role models.

✳ I never had a conscious thought of studying medicine until the age of twenty-five, but the scene at the moment I first had such a thought is engraved on my mind forever. A long, broad stretch of white sand, with the sea on one side and a gleaming white stucco hotel covered with scarlet bouganvellia on the other. The sky above was blue as only a Southern California sky could be on a clear day in the blazing sun (in the days before smog). The pungent scent of eucalyptus merged with the scent of the flowers and the sea. Laguna Beach. A far cry from the linoleumed halls and antiseptic aromas of a hospital, but it was in that very scene that something hitherto deeply hidden erupted. I stopped walking, turned to look at the sea, and said to myself, "I'm going to be a doctor." Nobody could have been more surprised than I was at that moment.

The whole idea was irrational and impossible. I had no money, and in the middle of the Depression no one else in the family had any money to help me either. I had no preparation. In college I had majored in German literature and history and had taken no science except the required course in biology during my freshman year. Afterward I had gone to live with my family in an exurban Connecticut farmhouse, studied shorthand and typing, and later moved back to New York, first to take a job as secretary in a copper company and later as junior copywriter in an advertising agency. Even after the emergence of that astonishing thought, I tried in a number of other ways to find myself, knowing that my life wasn't going where I wanted it to go. In spite of all that, within seven years of that day on Laguna Beach, I had graduated from medical school. That was forty-three years ago.

                 ✳ I have often asked others how they happened to get into the work by which they make a living and have obtained all sorts of answers. Sometimes it was chance—a job that just happened to be available at a particular time. Sometimes the influence of someone important in a person's life inspired a particular choice, or something developed from a hobby or long-term interest. All these answers have seemed reasonable and consistent with the circumstances of the person who gave them, but to me such reasons are both true and untrue. True on the surface, and true according to the conscious awareness of the person involved, but there is more to it. Why did that individual stay with that particular line of work after the emergency passed? To which of various possible alternatives did he or she respond? Why did I myself not stay with business or advertising? What combination of unrecognized thoughts and feelings came together in my unconscious mind at a particular moment to erupt as a wish to be something I had never even considered before that moment?

I can now give many rationalizations and realistic explanations for being where I am today, but I think the roots of my choice lie in the whole history and fabric of my life, starting with conception, or even before.

Perhaps more than some people, I tend to think in sensuous images, visual, olfactory, and tactile. I see the past, smell it, and feel it on my skin. The country place where I spent the first six summers of my life is exceedingly clear in my memory largely because I feel soft sand between my toes, taste the dusty leaves of sassafras grabbed from a roadside shrub as I rode in a four-seated buggy en route to the lake, smell the dust and leather, the sweat of the horses, and the dung that plopped from beneath their uplifted tails as we trotted along. I could describe every stick of furniture in that cottage and tell you its exact position in the room. It is still with me now as I write, and from such images I will reconstruct the early part of a life from which answers to these questions must come.

2 The World That Was, 1912—1929

Pictures from Childhood

PICTURES IN AN ALBUM   I have heard it said that a student of dianetics could remember riding on his daddy's sperm. My own memory does not reach that far back, although no doubt my daddy's sperm carried within it much of what I am today. But we cannot overlook the genes carried by the egg into which it plunged on a day in May 1911. A few years ago I saw a rerun of myself being interviewed on television after the publication of a book and reacted momentarily with a great sense of shock. There on the screen was my mother, looking just as I knew her before she returned to my father after twenty years of separation. I had been told throughout the years that I looked like her but had never before realized that it was true. I had also been told many times that I looked like my paternal grandmother, as did my father, both of his sisters, and my own sister. I dare say that is true too, because in many ways I feel myself to be a strange combination of my parents, in ways both contradictory and confusing. How much is due to genes? My parents were totally different kinds of people, and I suspect the confusion lies as much, if not more, in nurture as in nature.

Although some people think otherwise, I cannot believe that memory is carried in the genes. I do believe, however, that very soon after birth impressions occur that can remain locked up in the unconscious mind of an individual and emerge later as preverbal memories consisting of sensuous images. I have heard many people describe visual and auditory memories from the first few months of life, and I myself remember the scene left by a flood which occurred at our country place when I was nine months old, and frequently appeared in a recurrent dream of childhood. The tendency to think in such images usually fades as a child develops the capacity to use language and concepts built on words begin to form in the child's mind. However, the memories of some people retain a strong visual quality. This may be an inherited characteristic which is sometimes prominent in artists, although many people think it is the result of experiences in the earliest stages of life that fix a visual mode of thinking. In any case, memories from early childhood which appear as visual images usually represent emotionally charged events and interactions with people of particular significance in the child's development.

So it is with me. I can evoke a number of strong visual images from the first five or six years of life which I believe portray states of mind and attitudes that were gradually built into my character, forming the structure of what I later became. However, for most images from the very earliest months, which portray the emotional reactions of a very small child, I have to rely largely on baby pictures in a family album.

There have been times throughout my life when suddenly, for no apparent reason, an overwhelming feeling of depression hits me and sets up eddies in my head. At such moments I can neither think nor feel anything except lethargy and terrible sorrow. Without visible provocation, I used to burst into a flood of tears, as though something unseen had tapped into an underground well and brought up a gusher. Perhaps that metaphor relates to a childhood image of my body as a bag of flesh filled with blood—no concept of bones or inner organs— just blood that spurts out whenever you get pricked anywhere. That is the way I still sometimes think of my inner self—just a bag of tears, despite all those months of studying anatomy to discover what the body is like inside.

Heaven knows I've had my share of sadness and trauma, but there have been far more pleasure and interest in my life than grief. I have had successes in most of my undertakings, friends, lovers, and husbands—people who really mattered to me and I to them. I have achieved respect in my field, written books and received awards, and I live in comfort, surrounded by beauty. What feeds this underground well of sorrow, and why has it remained underground when on the surface there has always run a river of sparkling capacity to be active and enjoy? The source of the spring must lie very early in the experiences of life.

One can already see the dichotomy in two portraits of a three-year-old girl dressed in the finest voile, inset with lace. One is a happy, impish child, hands relaxed in her lap, laughing gleefully at whatever was going on in the photographic studio. The other has an incredibly sad little face, and although she holds a ball, there is no joy in her. She has on the same beautiful dress with its embroidered, lace-trimmed collar covering her shoulders; she is obviously in the same studio, on the same day, looking at the same photographer; but her face in repose is the face of a different child. Looking at this picture now makes me want to cry. Where did it come from, this sadness latent in a highly privileged and protected little girl? We have to go back still further.

In that family album are two portraits of a four-month-old baby. One shows a beautiful woman holding the child. She wears a long dressing gown of silk and lace, and a thick braid of hair encircles her head, which is tilted over her right shoulder as she gazes up at her infant with an adoring smile. The infant is held high, facing the photographer, almost at arm's length from the mother's body. Its fists are clenched, and on its face is an expression of abject terror. It is perfectly obvious that this infant, dressed in an elaborate long baby dress of the kind fashionable during that era, has every expectation of being dropped.

On the opposite page is the picture of another woman holding the same infant, who now wears an embroidered cape with a cap covering its little round head. The woman is dressed in a uniform representing the Boston hospital which, during that era of nannies, trained fresh-faced Irish lasses and German fräuleins such as this one to care for the young of American families who could afford baby nurses. Over a striped cotton dress with a stiff white collar she wears a voluminous white, bibbed apron also stiff with starch and, covering a knot of hair on the top of her head, a starched white mortarboard cap. The nurse also holds the baby facing the camera, but she holds it close to her body, and on her plain, kindly face is a look of calm. The baby is calm too, although its large round eyes stare warily at the camera.

In these pictures lie the clues—the roots of a duality in this child's approach to the world, the expectations of loving care and protection right alongside the uncertainty of achieving real love and security, which persisted for many years thereafter. Here is the nurturant nurse who carried out all the bodily care for this infant after her sixth week of life. There is the woman who wanted so much to be a good mother but could not manage to breastfeed the "accidental" child of her mid-thirties and had to turn her over to a stranger. It is obvious that she was terribly proud of that baby and would see to it that she had every advantage. But it is also obvious that by the age of four months the infant had already learned to sense limitations to the warmth available from that particular source. The pictures tell it all.

* Within this infant, donated by both her parents, are genes from the handsome people in this album, which begins with a portrait of my maternal grandfather as a curly-haired young man, later shown as a white-haired, clean-shaven man of the Edwardian era. He was a big businessman and, at the height of his powers, a high official of a railroad that practically owned the state of California. His stately wife, seen here in an elaborate Victorian gown, was the mother of six children and a leader of San Francisco society during the 1890s.

I had periodic contact with these maternal grandparents from my childhood well into adult life, although they lived far away and visits were few. I can remember events in which they had a part and recognize pictures of them at ages that corresponded with my early days. But the only images of them in my mind's eye are from the years when I was already an adult. I can picture their house, filled with yellow flowers, when I attended their golden wedding celebration at the age of nine, and the big dining room table surrounded by assembled relatives, before whom all the grandchildren had to recite poems of their own composition. But I cannot see them except as an old man with a white beard and a gentle little lady of nearly ninety in a red Spanish shawl, entertaining the family with stories of her Midwestern childhood. I think this tells something of their emotional impact on me, or lack of it.

What did they contribute to the person I became, these grandparents who meant so much to my mother for the whole of her life? I think first a sense of pride—pride in the prestige their name carried, at times when shame over my own father's mysterious activities was so threatening. I had been taught to honor them, and I did. I respected and revered them, and the fact that they were my grandparents helped to prop up my rather fragile sense of self-esteem during adolescence and even afterward. Secondly, a certain sense of material security. Where other people had to rely on loans, government grants, or Social Security, I relied on them to be there in emergencies and to pick up the pieces when my father's ventures threatened to leave us penniless. I sometimes felt able to take risks in my own career because I knew that I would probably inherit enough to keep me from want in my old age. They paid for my college education until I was able to qualify for a scholarship, and for this I am particularly grateful because I knew that my grandfather didn't believe in higher education for women. Last but not least, they bought for mother the comforting, beautiful Colonial farmhouse in Connecticut where even now, fifty years later, I have deep emotional roots. Life would have been a lot more difficult if they hadn't been there to back us up. I was grateful then, and am grateful now, but there was no real relationship between us until I was grown. Nothing of them went into my earliest beginnings except their genes.

With my paternal grandfather it was quite different. I retain a very vivid image of him from childhood, although I saw him only during the one summer he spent with us in Michigan when I was three, and not again until Mother and I spent an afternoon with him just before his death at the age of eighty-five. I was sixteen at the time and had just come up to the town where he lived in Northern California after a rather dreary summer in Los Angeles with my other grandparents. On the way up, we had stopped at an animal park where I had been allowed to hold a bobcat in my arms. When I now try to picture my grandfather at that time, all I can see is the bobcat. But I can picture him clearly as he was in his sixties on the farm because at that time I adored him. I ran to his cottage every morning and followed him around like a puppy. His picture in the album shows a youngish man whose pleasant expression is partly obscured by a large bushy mustache—a young man I never knew. But as I look at the picture, I can see a distinct resemblance to my first husband. I don't know if this is just a coincidence, but I doubt it. He was the first man for whom I felt love without a tinge of fear.

I never saw his wife, my paternal grandmother, who died of pneumonia before I was born, but in her portrait as a young woman it is easy to feel the piercing quality of her dark eyes and to see determination written all over her face. If there is one trait of character that permeated my father's family it was determination, and there is no doubt about where it came form. Of course, there must have been a lot of it in my mother's family too, and I certainly saw the fruits of it in my mother's lifelong persistence in maintaining the fantasy of a happy marriage against all seemingly rational evidence to the contrary. But my father's determination had a driven quality to it—an intensity that was overwhelming to all who knew him. He would fight for his rights against all odds, and he would fight to the death if necessary. I have it too, and at times it has stood me in good stead. Without it I don't think I could have worked with the kinds of patients with whom I have been most successful—those who require from their therapist an infinite, dogged persistence in overcoming seemingly hopeless resistances.

Whether qualities of that sort lie in the genes I don't know, but I suspect they do. As a pediatrician I have seen that kind of determination in certain newborn infants, and I have seen it in tiny toddlers of even the mildest, most easygoing parents. A baby picture of myself at the age of eighteen months leaves no doubt that I had it by that age.

A round-faced child with a ribbon around her head is dressed in lace-trimmed linen and high white buttoned shoes. She is seated on a chair, her arms held stiffly at her sides and one leg stuck out straight before her. Her lips are pressed together in an unsmiling stare of pure, stubborn defiance.

My mother used to tell me about the taking of that picture—how at first I had both legs stuck stiffly forward but finally, in response to her pleas and those of the photographer, I had slowly—very slowly—lowered one leg while continuing to stare at them without change of expression. I would compromise, but that is as far as I was prepared to go.

It has been like that most of my life, although as time went on, nurture added to nature. I can still hear my father's booming voice laying down the laws. "If you are wrong, don't be afraid to admit it, but if you are right, stick to your guns until you take the fort." How to be sure you were right—that was always a problem to me although it never seemed to bother him. He knew he was right at all times. However, I tried to follow that advice, and everything in my nature went along with it. Without that trait I don't think I would have made it through the hard years of adolescence and early adulthood. Although the overwhelming stubbornness of both parents was ever before my eyes as a negative role model, I think that trait was born in me, and I am glad it was.

Pictures in My Mind

Sometimes when I am listening to people tell about their problems, a picture comes into my mind. This picture often gives me a clue to what they are feeling at the moment, even when they themselves may be unaware of the feeling. By a mental process similar to that involved in forming dreams, I have condensed into a single symbolic image a number of the patient's associations which are tied together by a common emotional state. I have somehow connected them with experiences of my own where similar feelings were evoked and made an emotional association. Thus I can empathize with what is going on in them even before arriving at an intellectual formulation.

I believe that when memories from my own childhood appear in a strongly visual form, something similar occurs. Such memories, which carry a particular emotional charge, often symbolize the emotional states occurring at the time of the event visualized. For instance, from early childhood I have almost no visual memories of my sister, who was ten years older and took almost no direct part in my life at the time. My mother talked about her constantly, telling me at every age every detail of what my sister had said or done at the same age, and I know I idealized her for years. But the one clear image I have of her from my first five or six years tells the true story of my feelings. A little girl "jokingly" throws a mass of burrs into her older sister's heavy mane of black hair as her mother lovingly brushes it. It is all there—the years of concealed envy and resentment for her dominant place in my mother's affections.

So it is with most early events and places I see clearly in my mind's eye. They represent the quality of my relationships with significant people and my feelings about them in the period before I was seven and a half. That is the age at which I left the house where I was born and ended the so-called formative years.

✳ The house where I spent my early years was a gray stone townhouse—what some people call a row house— on the near North Side of Chicago. It was fairly small but solid and attractive, decorated outside with window boxes of bright flowers and inside with the Oriental rugs and solid mahogany furniture in vogue at the time. In the back was a large yard in which all the neighborhood children played. The street, once fashionable, was no longer so, but it was still "respectable" and for a time remained acceptable even to the few families on the block who considered themselves part of a fashionable world.

I can see the rooms of that house with photographic clarity, down to the exact placement of every chair and ornament. "Downstairs" represented my parents, sister and servants in the kitchen, who had a big part in my life. The whole third floor, consisting of two bedrooms and a large playroom, represented Fräulein, my brother, and me.

Fräulein was an unmarried woman in her mid-thirties, of peasant stock and recently arrived in this country, where she had had hospital training in Boston as a baby nurse. She had spent her early life in a small German village and, while working for us, was in the process of establishing American citizenship. She was stolid, unimaginative, and compulsively clean, but kindly, efficient, and devoted in carrying out her duties to me. Her sister, who became our cook for a while, owned a bakery in another area of the city where Fräulein often took me on her days off. Even now the smell of a bakery floods me with waves of nostalgia.

The person who carries out major bodily care of an infant becomes that child's psychological mother, whether that person is female or male. By the way their bodies are handled by a caretaker—the way they are held, fed, bathed, and spoken to—very young children sense the caretaker's attitudes toward them. Through that awareness, transmitted without words, they begin to develop their own feelings about themselves and their expectations of feelings that others will have toward them in the future. A child's relationship to the primary caretaker is one of the most important relationships in that child's life, no matter what comes later, and Fräulein was my primary caretaker.

Fraulein was my psychological mother.

I had another mother too, a loving mother who had a great influence on my development even during that early period. But it was Fräulein who fed me and bathed me and put me to bed. She was the one who took me for daily walks, showed me animals in the zoo, and helped me off and on with my galoshes and heavy knitted leggings when we entered the steamy flower house in the park. She read me bedtime stories, kissed me goodnight, and slept beside me in one of the two brass beds in the room we shared. She was my most constant companion for the first five years of my life, and it was in her language that I learned to communicate. She was the person who served as a source for my early identifications, and it was for this reason that I lost her rather abruptly at the age of five. Although I was told at the time that she was leaving because I was too old to have a nurse any more, Mother told me in later years that Fräulein was fired because I was even beginning to look like her. My mother could no longer tolerate her jealousy of the love I gave to Fräulein.

A little girl torn between love for two mothers, sensing their competitiveness—a little girl coming to know that the person she loved most was somehow inferior and her language laughable. A primarily German-speaking child in an English-speaking family. It is all condensed into a couple of images.

A small child stands on a staircase, looking down into a living room, where adults and a boy in a sailor suit look up. Under one arm the child clutches a stuffed white rabbit. I can see it very clearly. The little boy teases his baby sister by saying, "That's *my* bunny!" The little girl solemnly and firmly states, "That is your bunny *not!*" Everyone laughs. Fräulein is not in the picture, but she is there in that inverted word order and in the seldom-smiling little face. And she is there in the humiliation of feeling like an outsider in one's own family. No doubt I *was* beginning to look like her, and no doubt by then I knew that to be like her was somehow laughable and demeaning.

Another picture appears now. Mother and I are on one of the weekly excursions we take together in her little electric automobile and have stopped at the house of a dressmaker. Hanging on the rack is a spangled, sequin-covered, brightly colored child's dress that I covet with a deep passion. Right this moment I can feel how much I wanted that dress! Mother explained, of course, that it wasn't at all suitable for me—that probably it was the costume for a little actress. I'm sure I accepted that, as I accepted most of her explanations, but what I remember is the tone of voice in which she at first laughed and said, "There's the

Fräulein in you!" Contempt for Fräulein's flashy taste—the feather boa around her neck when she went for "days out," the tiny rhinestones in her pierced ears.

Mother never said anything against Fräulein to me. In fact once, later on, when she was complaining about my disloyalty to my father, she said, "I always thought one of the most admirable things about you was your loyalty to Fräulein." But I knew how she felt. I myself thought Fräulein was beautiful when she was dressed up and smelled lovely in her cheap violet perfume. Pink cheeks and white powdered skin. Perhaps she, more than anyone else, was responsible for the split in my mind between what "nice people" did and what was sensuously pleasurable. That, and the fact that flashy types often seemed to please my father, lipservice to the contrary.

Those two images represent the anguish of a small child caught in a clash of opposing social values between people she loved, and the ambivalence she felt toward the one considered inferior. However, all the *un*ambivalent feelings—all the joy of coziness and love and security of the nursery years—are condensed in a single image connected by association to a dramatic event in my later life.

A tiny child in gingham rompers and high black buttoned shoes sits on the lap of her nurse, almost lost in a billowing white apron. In the nurse's hand is a German edition of *Grimm's Fairy Tales* from which she reads, and on the table beside her is a lamp in the shape of a tree. I thought that lamp beautiful, perhaps because she had given it to me. Later I learned how she had often bought me elaborate presents that she could ill afford, for which my mother felt compelled to reimburse her. But at the time I only knew I loved that lamp as I loved other things she gave me—the rainbow-striped blanket she knitted and the huge doll crib lined in blue silk that would hold my entire family of teddy bears. I loved the twisted iron trunk of that lamp and the Tiffany glass shade all covered with green leaves. To me that lamp *was* Fräulein.

I found this out years later when, while driving along through the Black Forest, I suddenly felt an irresistible impulse to get out of the car and throw my arms passionately around the gnarled trunk of a giant tree. At that moment I almost believed that a woodcutter's cottage lay just around the bend, and I can still feel traces of the pain that poured out of me in a flood of tears. Sorrow over the loss of my nurse—love and sorrow that had been festering within me for over twenty years. At that moment it all came out—at least the part that ever *can* come out of an emotion so deeply buried at such an early age. Part of it, I'm sure, will never come out completely and is one trickle that will probably forever feed my underground well of tears. Other trickles flow from the residue of sorrow over each important loss in my life thereafter. Whenever I lose a loved one, people, animals, or beloved places, something plugs into that pool of tears and I weep for all the lost ones together with equal intensity. Losing them makes them all one to me.

Early loss of important love objects causes a lot of problems for a lot of my patients. I know just what it feels like.

✳ My brother was five years older than I, already attending school by the time I became conscious of him, but he was a very important figure in my early life. In those days I thought my feelings toward him were pure hatred, although I can now see how mixed they were. I hated him for his constant teasing and deeply resented the fact that my mother's usual response was to tell me it was "all in fun" and I shouldn't let it bother me. It *did* bother me, and although I cannot remember that he ever hurt me physically, he certainly was a constant source of torment and anxiety.

However, there were many times when we played together quite happily in his big room down the hall from mine. I can see it now— the cabinets full of games and a large table by the window holding fascinating small wooden boxes and bottles full of multi-colored crystals and liquids in his chemistry set. We did magic tricks together and played geography board games. We named our respective goldfish "Acapulco" and "Manzanillo," and in the year 1917, we created "war books."

Those war books have a particular place in my memory, and I still regret that they were among the treasures lost in later years when storage bills could not be paid. They seemed very exciting, containing a child's view of World War I—posters of Red Cross nurses and Uncle Sam saying "I want *You!*" Liberty bonds, war savings stamps, and sheets from the rotogravure each week showing the faces of soldiers lost in no-man's-land. We worked on those books together, and in later years we both longed to see them again. Of course mine was a joke compared to his, filled largely by his cast-offs and duplicates. It would have looked like nothing. Perhaps that's why I see the books so clearly. They were symbolic of everything of his that was so much bigger and better than mine. Like his trench in the backyard, where we played at "going over the top." I can see it too—his trench over his head in depth, mine much shallower because Mother was afraid it would cave in on me. Why wouldn't *his* trench cave in? Things like that wouldn't happen to a boy, I suppose, although they probably *would* happen to a little girl trying to keep up. My Freudian colleagues will remind me that these are the usual images representing penis envy in a little girl, but I'll tell *you* that a little girl has a lot more to envy than a penis in a brother five years older and a lot stronger.

To sum it all up, I see the picture of a ten- or eleven-year-old-boy on crutches in the backyard, recouperating from a broken leg, and a little girl in a checked gingham dress "accidentally" pushing him over. That picture is accompanied by a feeling of guilt. What if I had seriously injured him again, just as he was getting to the point when he could again tease and torment me? What if something *I* did, without consciously meaning to, had damaged him for the rest of his life? I have wondered that so many times, about so many aspects of our relationship to each other and to our parents. What *did* it do to him when I replaced him as our father's favorite because I seemed to have capabilities that our father had wanted in a *son?* Waves of guilt still wash over me occasionally when I think that my brother's damaged life might in fact have had something to do with the birth of a sister whose baby carriage he, in turn, had "accidentally" pushed off a high porch when she was an infant.

Many symptoms brought to a psychiatrist for understanding have at their core envy and anger toward important people in their lives, and the guilt for such feelings. I've been there, and I know what that feels like too.

✳ As I think of him now, my father was a strange combination of opposing traits. On the one hand, he was a hard-driving, ruthless businessman, autocratic and egocentric. He had been second in command at two of the most powerful newspapers in the country and left them largely because he couldn't bear being second in command to anyone. However, when he founded his own business, it was at least partly to satisfy another side of his character, the idealist and dreamer who actually came close to making some of his wildest fantasies real.

His was one of the first cooperative grocery businesses in the country, founded with the idea that a man could make enormous profits while still improving the lot of the "little guy." To him, everyone who wasn't as enterprising and powerful as he was a little guy, and his intention was to give this little guy better goods at a cheaper price while still making a bundle for himself. Unfortunately, this constituted a threat to others in the produce business of that hog-butchering, meat-packing metropolis of the world and got him into a lot of trouble beginning during my early childhood. Of course, I didn't know anything about all that.

I did know that he had been poor in his youth and wanted his children to have everything he hadn't had. But he also wanted us to realize that everyone didn't live as we did. It worried him that we had so little contact with people from other walks of life, and it was partly for this reason that throughout the summers we spent on our on farm in Michigan, he arranged to have small groups of teenage factory workers from Chicago visit for two weeks at a time. I was only four or five but can still see a girl with long black braids and a red sweater who told me stories about the textile factory where she worked. All day long it was her job to break the thread and separate each finished garment from the assembly line, and sometimes toward the end of the day she would faint from the monotony and tedium. That made a big impression on me. She was afraid of the cows and of sounds the owls made at night, but she ran with us through the woods and collected eggs with us in the chicken yard. Whether it was a good experience for her I don't know, but it was good for us. My father was quite right about that.

At home he was boisterous, insensitive, and became exceedingly nervous if anyone crossed him, but to me he was "Daddy" who was "away at business" most of the time and was always kind to me.

I picture him only in the living and dining rooms of that house and don't believe I ever saw him above the first floor. He certainly never invaded my territory on the third floor, and I never descended to the second until after he had left for work. Upstairs was my domain, downstairs the parental domain, which was separate from my own geographically as it was emotionally. There was no crawling into the parental bed on a Sunday morning; no bursting in on nudity or urination, as so many women seem to remember doing in their childhood; no catching anyone in the "primal scene." I had my fantasies, like everyone else, but even after many years of psychoanalysis I say with some assurance that I never saw my father other than fully clothed—that is, not only with his pants on but also with a starched, wing-collared shirt, coat, and tie, even on the hottest days of summer. His shiny black high-buttoned shoes were polished every day, too. That was his concept of the way a "gentleman" appeared before "ladies"—even in his own castle, where two of the ladies were fifteen and five, respectively.

What images I have of him are of his literally blowing into the living room in a blast of cold air from outside, hanging his coat in a large armoire at the foot of the stairs, and proceeding almost immediately to the dining room, where he presided over a nightly scene of mayhem. I can see him now as he tells us all to "sit up straight" before he finishes sitting down. We children immediately slump in our seats as a reflex response to his order, thereby setting off a minor war between him and us. However, by the time I could see that, I was older and had joined my siblings in their battle against him. In the earlier period, my feelings about him were good.

Twice a year he took us on an excursion to Riverview, an amusement park, which I anticipated eagerly throughout the year. And almost every evening, before it was time for Fräulein to sweep me off to the nursery, he reluctantly but faithfully played cards with us, "Bunco" and "Pit"—the big event of the day. "Pit" was a game about the stock market, with bulls and bears. All I can remember about "Bunco" is the figure of a policeman on one of the cards. If it turned up in your hand you could yell "Stop!" to anyone who was having a turn and take over the play yourself. How I loved that! I so seldom had a chance to say "Stop!" to anyone.

Once I nagged my father to tell me what I was going to get for Christmas. It was supposed to be a surprise, of course, but I guess he thought I'd never be able to figure it out if he scrambled up all the letters of "kitchen cabinet"—a real but small cabinet filled with tiny sample packages of all sorts of foods which were sent out as advertisements. I was not yet six, but I solved the puzzle, to everyone's amazement. Perhaps that was the beginning of my interest in anagrams and word games, but I know that by giving me a task supposedly beyond my ability my father gave me something far more important. He gave me the first awareness that I was bright and might be able to be somebody in our family after all.

He also spoiled me by his obvious favoritism and gave me a load of guilt to carry for the rest of my life. The beef juice! It remained a bone of contention between me and my brother even after we were adults, and he never quite forgave me for getting it all those years. Platter juice from a roast of beef was supposedly the prerogative of the baby in the family. Served in one of Mother's engagement cups, green porcelain with pink roses, it went to my sister until my brother took over five years later, and to him until I came along. After that it was mine, and nobody else came along to take it away from me. I suspect that my father took a certain amount of satisfaction from my brother's frustration, thinking, I suppose, that he was teaching him to be "a man." I, blissfully unaware of the envy and resentment, took it as my due and relished every drop. Of course now I can hardly smell the juice from a roast without being bathed in guilt.

In view of the anger I felt toward my father later in life, it surprises me that I took to heart so much of what he said. He wasn't one to talk *with* people; he *told* them and orated to them and didn't really expect any response except agreement and obedience. "Think for yourself!" he would say, which could be translated to mean "Figure things out so that you will see them my way." I understood that later, but at the time I took the words at face value, not realizing that they didn't fit the music. Even now hardly a day passes that I don't hear some of his words. The mark of his personality is stamped indelibly on mine, because, regardless of what happened later, I loved him at a time that really mattered in my development.

✳ My mother was a sweet and gentle soul, raised in the tradition of noblesse oblige. Her major aim in life was to be a good wife, a good mother, and a good Christian woman. She did everything in her power to be all three, devoting herself to what she felt to be in the best interests of her husband and children while also working for charitable causes. She paid her servants better than average wages and gave them both comfortable and attractive living quarters, a practice that was not widespread among her acquaintances. Unlike many women of her class and condition, Mother did not believe in taking advantage of "less fortunate" people. She despised there of her peers who were "purse proud," making scathing remarks about women she knew who cut the buttons off their expensive dresses before giving them to the poor. She was polite to everyone, rich or poor, and did her best to help those in need.

If anyone had told my mother that she was a snob she would have been horrified. She didn't believe in snobbery and often inveighed against it. But she was a snob all the same, along with a lot of other people who do not recognize themselves as such. She knew, of course, that many respectable people were not listed in the Social Register, but they were in an orbit that seldom crossed hers, and "cheap people" were in another galaxy. This did not include the "simple" people who were poor merely because they lacked the vision and enterprise that had enabled my father to extricate himself from poverty. Such people were "good" but remote from her life. Cheap people were loud and flashy and irresponsible about other people's property, and for them she had no sympathy at all.

Mother took the values of her class for granted and never quite realized that the privileged people with whom she had always associated were a tiny segment of the population outside the mainstream of American society. I believe that to her "Society" meant the socially prominent families of successful big-business and professional men from white, Anglo-Saxon, Protestant communities in major metropolitan areas. I don't think she really knew that in these same cities there were many groups of well-educated, cultured, and refined people who did not belong to Society and did not particularly want to. It never crossed her mind that there might be "nice people" fully as privileged as those belonging to Society who might actually choose to send their children to schools, dancing schools, and summer places other than those considered "best" in her world. She could sympathize with anyone who couldn't afford these "advantages," but that any intelligent people existed who might not want the kind of life she wanted for herself and her children was a concept outside her experience.

Mother wanted her children to have the best of everything—the advantages that would enable them to fit in with the kind of people who belonged to the Society she knew—and she did all she could to give it to them, often at great personal sacrifice. She was as kind and lovable a woman as she set out to be—one who could also be lively and amusing in a rather childlike way and, when the chips were down, could show both courage and resourcefulness. However, she was also in many ways an extremely naive and stubborn woman, who carried to her death the conviction that if you believe something firmly enough, you can make it true. That was her undoing.

A small child, of course, knows nothing about the subtleties of her parent's character. To me, this beautiful, kindly, mixed-up lady was simply "Mother." *My* mother. In thinking about her, the first image that comes to mind is not of her at all but of a giant Christmas tree, its tip touching a high ceiling. A little girl looks with awe at its grandeur—the strings of cranberries, popcorn, and tinsel, the gilded walnut shells with crêpe paper fringes, the striped candy canes and tiny apples, the gingerbread men and stars. Did people have glass balls in those days? I don't see any on that tree; only hundreds of little candles, lighted only on Christmas Day. I guess people didn't worry so much then about fire hazards. As I look back, the few memories I have of active happiness in early childhood are centered around Christmas, and Christmas was Mother. She was the one who made it happen. She went all-out to make it good, and it was.

In my earliest years, the tree was brought to the playroom by Santa Claus, who decorated it during the night. Later it was in the living room, but we still had to wait until Christmas morning to see it. We woke at dawn, if we had slept at all, and found our stockings on the bedpost to play with until noises from downstairs indicated that our parents were awake. The stockings were always glorious—not just our own little socks stuffed with toys but large ones made of net or felt. The contents varied from year to year but always included a few traditional things. No matter what else was in it, each stocking always had a tangerine in the toe and a liberal supply of lichee nuts throughout. I can see myself lying in bed, looking at my stocking with half-closed eyes in the gray of earliest morning, trying to figure out what was in it from the shape of the bulges—containing my curiosity and excitement as long as possible before pouncing.

Then there was Mother's own little table-sized tree on Christmas Eve, loaded with little joke objects and limericks about each member of the family. Even after we were adult we didn't let her stop fixing that tree, and I can still experience the keen anticipation with which I waited for it—my hope that *this* year my joke would be a little bit more personal. Of course Mother didn't really *know* much about the minutiae of my daily life because I spent my life with Fräulein. She couldn't make the kinds of joke about me that she did about the others, but each year I hoped anew and tried to suppress my disappointment. Odd, isn't it, that I, who have almost total recall for the words and music of almost every popular song written since the Victorian era and can still recite a French poem I learned in the first grade, can't remember a single limerick that Mother wrote about me in all those years?

Other things disappointed me too. My toys, no matter how big and beautiful, were never quite as good as those of a friend whom I usually visited right after Christmas. But nobody can be blamed for that. If I was always comparing what I got to what others were given, the fault lay in my way of looking at the world and not in any real deprivation.

I have talked with many people who were truly deprived of material necessities in childhood and I sometimes feel ashamed that they seem to have come to terms with their deprivation far better than I, who had every possession a child could possibly want. It has been surprising to me that many such people have been able to understand, often far better than those who have never suffered any deprivation, that a rich child can feel as deprived as a poor one. The feeling is so relative to expectations, isn't it?—so much a matter of contrast between what one has and what one has been taught to want, between aspiration and achievement. More than that, material possessions have so often become symbols reflecting feelings about relationships in a child's life that are lacking in some essential ingredient, or seem to be.

Christmas, more than any other time in the year, was a time of fun and family togetherness. It was a time when I felt I really belonged to the family, and there weren't too many times like that. There is a picture in the family album of Mother and my two siblings seated at the dining room table. I knew very well that it had been taken before I was born, but this didn't stop me from asking over and over, "Where was *I*, Mother?" All her reasonable answers never answered the real question or took away the persistent feeling of being outside that threesome.

I see them now from the doorway of a cabin on the night boat to Michigan. It had been a stormy night on the lake, and the scene before me was one of chaos. Mother had made a bed of sorts for herself on the floor, while in the double bunk were two pale, miserable children who had spent the night vomiting all over the bed. Fräulein and I had come from our own neat, comfortable cabin, where nobody had been seasick. We stood there looking at them, and they looked at us. On all those ghastly, unhappy faces was a look of incredible envy for two clean, well-breakfasted souls ready for a walk around the deck, but as I look at that scene now, I feel again the sweep of loneliness that I felt then and at almost every other time I witnessed their togetherness.

Why did I never feel a part of that tight little group even when I actually was a part of it? After the earliest nursery years I was with them all quite often—at lunch, where Mother read the Oz books and I stood by her side following the words as she read. That was how I learned to read at an early age, and it should be a memory that gives me great satisfaction. At lunch I was also an active participant in the "table manners game." Each of us had before our place a glass filled with pennies, and whenever someone transgressed, a penny passed from his or her glass to Mother's empty one. I became quite adept at catching others when they slipped and eagerly preserved my own hoard of riches. It was in the spirit of fun and exciting competition that we learned table manners, and there were many times that the *four* of us shared laughter and good times. Mother had a childlike sense of humor and was full of riddles, puns, and little games to amuse children. I remember all those good times, but they just didn't register emotionally. What did register was the feeling of never being either quite in or quite out of the group—a feeling that was reinforced later by other situations and became a real handicap. I never for a moment during my childhood doubted that my mother loved me. I was quite conscious of feeling that she loved my siblings better, although I knew she loved me too and would always serve my best interests as she saw them. But I didn't realize that my feeling that anything I had wasn't quite as good as what others had, that in any group I would be odd man out, had anything to do with her. How could a child know that feelings about the better toy or admittance to the inner circle had anything to do with feelings about a mother's love?

In spite of all the ups and downs, I loved my mother throughout my life. As a child I wanted to be near her whenever I could. Why is it that when I try to place her in the rooms of that house the images are not of her but of things closely associated with her in my mind, like Christmas and the bureau in her bedroom? Its top was just at my eye level, covered with ruby glass bottles and silver-handled utensils, brushes, nail files, chamois nail buffers and button hooks. (What child today would recognize a button hook? But there it was among the other things on the embroidered bureau scarf, an essential tool in that era of high-buttoned shoes and kid gloves to the elbow.) I can remember the exquisite pleasure of looking through her drawers—piles of dainty chiffon and lace interspersed, with balls of lavender and sachet and the delicate spotted veils that ladies of the era wore drawn across their faces. I can remember so many things about her, but I can't see her. I picture her clearly only in the one room to which she almost never came, the playroom.

A little girl in a pink chiffon dress holds in her hand a cracked glass alcohol lamp discarded from her brother's chemistry set. Somehow she has managed to fill it, spilling a lot on her dress. I don't see her light the match, but I see the flames rising and hear her frantic cries as she tries to beat at them with her hands. Then I see Mother, miraculously plunging through the door, having recognized the peculiar quality of those cries and flown up two flights of stairs to wrap her baby in a rug and extinguish the flames. She saved me from permanent scarring then and from a lot of other miseries later. Perhaps the charge on that memory is not the terror and pain but the feeling that in an emergency my mother actually could perceive the intensity of my distress and come flying to the rescue. It happened only in an emergency, I think, but perhaps it was only at such times that I cried loud enough to let her hear. I knew she wanted me to be happy and spent most of my life protecting her from the knowledge that it wasn't always so.

❋ The little girl that I was on Deming Place lived in a world of ambivalent relationships—a world in which privilege, luxury, and love were never sufficient to overcome feelings of inferiority, deprivation, and exclusion. She was a high-strung child, pampered by a doting nurse, titillated by a father who showed favoritism and admiration for moments without continuity, and tormented by an older brother whose envy and resentment were unrecognized and ignored by her mother. She loved two mothers whose competitiveness stretched her loyalties and loaded her with guilt no matter which way she turned. In spite of all the warmth and pleasure she got from her own mother, she could never really reach her. That was a little girl with lots of problems to solve.

In her playroom is a tall cabinet-dollhouse whose rooms are furnished with delicate reproductions of Victorian furniture. It is the home of a doll family, and the little girl stands before it, anxiously talking to herself as she moves the dolls and furniture around from room to room. She keeps readjusting the environment for those dolls but never seems satisfied with the results. After a while, though, the intensity of the activity decreases, the anxiety fades, and she turns to go about other business. She has, for the moment, worked out some inner struggle through a form of therapeutic play, just as she later did with paper dolls, and as I still do by moving the furniture around in my living room. Before she left the house on Deming Place and entered into a whole new phase of existence, she had developed a method for handling periods of anxiety that stayed with her for a lifetime.

That little girl was never aware of what bothered her so much but, as small children frequently can, was able to work through some of her feelings in play without ever becoming conscious of them. She did not think of herself as unhappy or conflicted but took it for granted that her parents loved her as they said they did. The ability to contact deeper level of feeling went underground, and a growing girl lost contact with the child she had been. Nearly thirty years later, however, that child was resurrected by one of those mysterious connections between the present and the buried past which cause the eruption of hitherto unsuspected ideas. On that day a pediatrician who had until a few moments earlier been sitting in a hospital room watching the play of an eight-year-old boy suddenly stopped in the middle of the hall and said "Eureka!" Just as on a sunny California beach over ten years earlier she had said, "I'm going to be a doctor," she now said "I'm going to be a psychiatrist!" She said it with a feeling of absolute conviction, and from that time on, never changed her mind again.

✳ The seven and a half years I spent on Deming Place amounted to the longest span of time I lived anywhere until I married, over thirty years later. Within the next five years I had ten different addresses, not counting summer places, which also changed from year to year after my first six years in Michigan. Leaving the house on Deming Place was only one of the upheavals that took place in the life of our family, and for me it marked the end of all continuity except at school.

In 1919 my sister was seventeen. Principally for her sake, Mother felt it essential for all of us to move away from a rapidly declining neighborhood into a "downtown" world along Lake Shore Drive, so the house was sold in June, and we summered in Winnetka.

My memories of that summer are not of Ravinia, although I did see "The House that Jack Built" in that lovely open-air summer theater. The images I have are of myself learning to ride a bicycle and of our dog, Dicky, who was run over by a car and received a spinal injury resulting in priapism that first made me aware of penises. We had to leave him with friends at the end of the summer because we were to be in a hotel for a while, and when I heard later that he had run away trying to find us, my heart nearly broke. I had lost my nurse, and I had lost my home. Now we had "abandoned" Dicky, and he couldn't bear it. Neither could I. I see that little beagle still, running along the railroad track where he had last seen his family disappearing on a train, and my eyes are full of tears as I write. That image has plugged into the underground pool.

From the hotel where we spent the next month or so I have only one clear memory—one that represents the growing anxiety which I was beginning to relate to my father.

I believe that my father was an essentially good-hearted man who never meant to hurt anyone and was always distressed when he found that he inadvertently had. But there was a streak of sadism in him, which manifested itself in some rather questionable jokes. On one occasion, he brought home to my brother and me two rather elaborately wrapped presents, one big and one little, giving my brother first choice between them. When my brother chose the bigger one, as it was inevitable that he would, it had nothing significant in it. Mine was something quite nice, as I recall, which did nothing to improve relations between me and my brother. Nor did it do much to teach my brother about the pitfalls of greed, which was probably the intent.

While we were staying at that hotel, it was my father's job to wake us in the morning, as he did by jocularly singing, "It's music to the daddy's ears to hear the children squeal" while he jerked back our covers. This was "all in fun," but I faced it with such dread each morning that I finally could bear it no longer and greeted him by vomiting all over the bed. He never did it again, of course, and was abjectly sorry, but the image of that little girl cowering under the covers in terror of having them yanked off has never left me. Don't ask my Freudian friends what that was all about!

That fall my sister went to school in Italy. In the spring, Mother went to pick her up and spent three months traveling in Europe; my brother and I stayed in an apartment on Walton Place with our father and one of his former secretaries to take care of us. I battled with that woman constantly for the whole three months. That was the period in which paper dolls replaced my dollhouse as a therapy center, and by the time Mother returned at last, my equilibrium was at least partly restored. Daddy took me to New York to meet them at the boat, and almost as soon as we returned it was time to set off for a summer in Santa Barbara at the time of our grandparents' golden wedding anniversary.

So it went, one change after another. The next year we rented a big, beautiful apartment full of Louis Quinze antiques on Lake Shore Drive— a place that was right on the lake then but has since found itself inland, lost among huge hotels and condominiums. It was from there that my mother and I fled to Canada for a couple of months to avoid her involvement in my father's business troubles, and it was from there that my sister was married. I have lots of memories from that period, many of them good, but the only thing that made a lasting impression was that our much loved Pekingese was blown into the street and killed by a car on the stormy morning of my sister's wedding.

The wedding was in April, followed by a summer at the fifth resort we had tried since giving up the Michigan farm. Why we never returned anywhere for a second summer I don't know, but I really didn't care, because I had already discovered that I had no trouble making at least a few friends to swim and play croquet with. The one I remember from that summer was the only child of a man who had just struck oil in Oklahoma. Her mother wore a diamond the size of a pecan, and she herself had shoes dyed to match each of her dresses. They were nice, friendly people, and I've often wondered what happened to them. They were the only people from all those resorts that I remember at all.

By this time I was about to start seventh grade. My sister was gone, living in Connecticut; my brother was at boarding school in the East. We had moved into yet another, bigger apartment, with our own furniture out of storage, and it looked as though we might finally be settling down again. All hell had been breaking loose in my father's business life for the past year or more, and there had been screaming headlines about it in all the newspapers, which distressed my mother and sister beyond description. But none of this really touched me. I knew about it and knew that everyone in the family was in an uproar all the time, but it didn't affect my life at school or my relationships with my friends, which was what mattered to me. I had been to the same school since the first grade, had the same friends from year to year, and knew just which teachers and activities to expect next. I was very much involved in it all and was having a wonderful time. School was, in fact, the center of my life, until the bomb exploded. One day Mother told me she knew I was going to be sad, but certain things had been decided and there was nothing anyone could do about it. I had luckily been admitted to one of the finest day schools in the country, and within a month she and I would be moving East for good. I felt quite numb and didn't say a word.

Since losing my nurse and the home of my early childhood, I had lost two much loved dogs. Within four years I had lived in five different "homes," had gone to five different summer places, and had seen my siblings move out of my life. I had managed to remain unaffected because there was continuity in my school experience. Now that was to end also.

I was to leave the schoolhouse where my sister, as a departing senior, had planted ivy to cover the walls. I was to leave the friends with whom I had been in daily contact for six out of my eleven years, and I was to leave Chicago. I was to leave the lakefront where I had bicycled to school for the past four years—Michigan Boulevard, Sheridan Drive, and the Oak Street beach—Lincoln Park and the statues of civic leaders whose bronze laps I had polished with my own rear end. There would be no more twice-yearly trips to buy new shoes at Marshall Field, no more Field Days with three-legged races and lunchboxes holding the first fresh cherries of spring. There would, in fact, be no more of anything I had ever known. I was to leave my school, my city—and my father. It was too much, but nevertheless, in November 1923, just before my twelfth birthday, Mother and I took a train for New York and settled down in yet another apartment. My childhood was over.

I had no way of knowing that leaving all that behind was the best thing that had ever happened to me.

Preadolescence

Where is the New York I knew in the 1920s? Most of it seems to have disappeared along with the way of life we had before the Crash. A few years ago I returned there for the first time in many years, to attend a psychiatric meeting that happened to coincide with my fiftieth Brearley School reunion. The life I had led in New York during my teens and twenties had been sharply divided into three distinct periods, each connected with a different part of the city, but on this visit the impending reunion had thrown me back to a temporary state of nostalgia for the earliest of these. In that mood, I decided to revisit familiar places of my early youth and found with a sense of shock that most of them were gone. Almost without exception, even the buildings associated with that part of my life have been torn down.

Midtown Park Avenue, where 375 used to be, is now a forest of giant commercial structures. When I lived there, the avenue had a real park down the middle, site of the annual Park Avenue Fair, but there has been nothing left of that for forty years. The Racquet Club remains, its imposing façade now dwarfed between two huge piles of steel and glass, but the apartment house across the street, from which we looked down on it, has given way to the Seagram Building, with its foyers and fountains. The old Savoy Hotel on Fifth Avenue, where Mother and I spent six months, has been swallowed up by a behemoth monument to General Motors, along with all the little shops we used to patronize, and an apartment house now stands in place of our red brick, white-trimmed schoolhouse, where a young doctor named Ben Spock used to examine us after epidemics of measles and chicken pox. The old Ritz Carlton Hotel where we danced, the lot on Fifth Avenue and 102nd Street where our school held a Saturday morning playground, these are gone too, along with heaven only knows what other landmarks of fifty years ago. I wonder if the person I was has disappeared as completely as the environment in which I spent my early teens.

Recently, while cleaning out an old file, I came upon a little book hardly larger than a block of postage stamps. It was a diary, written in pencil faithfully throughout the year. This little book, given to me on my thirteenth birthday in early January 1925, gives a play-by-play account of what I thought and did every day of that year, and although no page contains more than forty words, it brings back to me a clear picture of a whole preadolescent period lasting four years or more. Seen from the perspective of today, this moratorium between childhood and adolescence lasted longer than it should have, and I find myself laughing at the innocence one wouldn't find in a ten-year-old today, but whether this is better or worse I am not prepared to say. I can say that the four years of that period were very, very full, and I look back on them as some of the most important in my whole life.

In these pages I can see clear evidence of the split that had been widening throughout the years—a split between the lively, active, intellectually stimulated and often rather hysterically overexcited girl who enjoyed life and carried out endless pranks among her classmates and teachers, and the quiet, withdrawn, openly frustrated girl whose home life was a constant source of anxiety and who spent every moment of her spare time either reading or going to the movies. How many images it evokes!

I see myself on that first day in my new school, rolling up my eyes and making a funny face to delight my classmates as the teacher introduced me. I could immediately see that I was "in" as the class clown and for the next four years did my best to live up to that image. Disrupting study hall with funny notes passed surreptitiously—disrupting classes by getting everyone to wear four or five glass bracelets and all erasing together on signal—disrupting the whole school by organizing the distribution of sneezing powder throughout the assembly hall. I still consider that the greatest organizational triumph of my life and love to think about what a great executive I might have become. Why the school tolerated me as well as it did is still something of a mystery.

I think at least part of the answer is that Brearley probably saw me as a "spirited" but essentially winsome and affectionate little girl who, in spite of her occasional bursts of deviltry and disruptiveness, was trying hard to be loved. In later years, while consulting with school-teachers from many different kinds of schools, it became obvious to me that a child who creates this kind of image is frequently forgiven a good deal by well-meaning adults, just as I was. The value of such an image decreases as time goes on, but I think I retained it pretty far into my adolescence, and it served me well. I apparently appealed to motherly women who recognized that I was hungry for mothering but was sensitive enough not to overdo the demand for it. I think those kindly women saw that being an enfant terrible was just a game—an attempt to get attention without meaning any real harm. The fact that I was also a good student and athlete didn't hurt any either. At that time and in that place, I was not the rebel I later became, and I think the faculty knew how much I needed an outlet for some of the frustration at home. They were a highly dedicated group of people in what was to me an intellectually stimulating and nurturant school.

Hardly a day passes that I haven't had occasion to be thankful for the quality of my education and of those who taught me. Lots of the so-called advantages given me turned out not to be advantages, but most of the schools I was privileged to attend both saved my life and were my life until I was grown. I had acquired a good foundation for learning before ever leaving Chicago—good study habits and an appreciation for the value of doing well. I could read at quite an advanced level and spell both *disappoint* and *disappear* without doubling the *s* or singling the *p.* I could write a decent composition neatly in ink without splutters and splotches, do almost anything in the fractions, and read simple stories in French. I knew all about Vikings and knights in armor and the life within a medieval castle, understood the function of chlorophyll, and had watched beans sprout their roots and leaves when placed between wet blotting paper and the side of a drinking glass. In short, I had completed a solid sixth-grade curriculum at the Girls' Latin School in English, history, math, general science, and foreign language, had done well and enjoyed it.

However, Brearley was different. I suppose by today's criteria it would be considered a traditional school, with high expectations and strict standards. When a paper was due it was due, and no excuses were accepted for handing it in late. We had lots of homework, lots of required outside reading, and every single month we had to learn, and recite to the class, one long poem and two short poems from an assigned list. We groaned, but we liked it. It was tough, but in that atmosphere learning became exciting, and what we learned stayed with us.

By the standards of that day Brearley was a progressive school where we got a lot of our education through making and doing. At this moment I can see the illuminated initial and medieval lettering on parchment paper that took me hours of creative effort. I remember my version of my own "Odyssey" written in the style of Homer. While walking in the country on a brisk New England fall day I remember "Oh world, I cannot hold thee close enough," and in times of stress I "thank whatever gods may be for my indomitable soul." Above all, I thank those gods for Elizabeth Littell, the science teacher who infected everyone in the class with genuine excitement over every little amoeba on every little slide. I think that she, probably more than anyone else, determined the course of my future.

A good part of my professional work has involved consulting with people in other professions which have an impact on people's mental health, such as psychiatrists, psychologists, social workers, teachers, and nurses. A good part of their professional work has involved dealing with disturbed families whose children are suffering from a traumatic environment. Often I am asked "What can we do for children exposed to disturbing influences?" My heartfelt answer usually is, "Do everything in your power to supply for these children adequate surrogates outside the home. Help them to find kind, sensible adults who will dilute the influence of the family and furnish healthier role models. Often that is the best anyone can do."

The science teacher of my preadolescent years became such a surrogate for me. She was a lady and a scientist, dedicated to the discovery of truth. She was the perfect role model for me, and my wish to identify with her as a lady who could also be a socially useful and productive person was a precursor of my later admiration for Mrs. Roosevelt, who had the same quality.

I saw in her a woman of charm and humor, who behaved with dignity and good breeding while dedicating herself fully and enthusiastically to useful work. She was a warm-hearted, sensitive woman who liked young people and treated them with respect, and she made me respect myself by taking an interest in my welfare. I was a hellion in that school, and most of the teachers didn't know quite what to do about me. She knew, however, instinctively and, I believe, through empathy. Many times when I was thrown out of class for giggling or making a stir, she neither preached nor moralized but invited me to the lab, where we did chemistry problems together for fun. If I had a free period that corresponded with one of hers, I was welcome to come for a talk, and talk I did into her sympathetic, non-judgmental ear. In later years I told her that she had been my "child therapist" and that I would have gone down the drain without her. She just laughed and said, "Nonsense! There was nothing the matter with you. All you needed was somebody to talk to." She was wrong about that, but I didn't know it then.

From her I learned that you can be a womanly woman and still use your mind—that "nice people" can belong to a broader world than Society and approach their world rationally without losing their capacity to have emotions. When she said, "Think for yourself," I came to know that she meant it, believing that people should value their own observations and draw their own conclusions before resorting to theories from books. I learned that from her in an atmosphere of friendship and caring, and it has become the cornerstone of my approach to education.

Would that every child in these troublesome days of overcrowded schools and inadequate curricula could find even one such teacher in the whole course of his or her education. What a difference it would make!

During that period I was having a rough time tolerating my life at home. When we left Chicago, the plan had been for my father to transfer his business affairs to the East and rejoin the family, but it never happened, and my mother became increasingly perturbed. For the first year or two he turned up fairly frequently for a day or two, full of promises, but soon it became obvious to everyone except my mother that he just wasn't coming to stay. I myself was very glad about that. Whenever he did come, the tension in our otherwise quiet household reached an unbearable pitch.

Ever since the beginning of his business troubles, my father had become increasingly nervous and upset—bombastically dictatorial, his pounding voice constantly nagging over every little thing that disturbed him. For me this was almost intolerable, producing such a feeling of tension that I expected to explode. In the middle of one argument I rushed from the dinner table, locked myself in my room, and, stuffing my pillow in my mouth, bit into it until a shower of feathers erupted like snow and flew all over the room. Later I told my one confidante that living with my father was like having a jackhammer in the room, although of course neither of us recognized what I was saying. If anyone had suggested that there was anything erotic in my rageful excitement I would been dumbfounded. All I knew was that I hated him—hated what he was doing to my mother and dreaded his visits. However, living on a day-to-day basis with my mother and seeing how his absence affected her filled me with guilt for such feelings.

After all those years of wanting my mother to myself, I was now the almost sole companion of a highly anxious religious fanatic who increasingly moralized, rationalized, and frantically tried to reassure herself that everything was as good and beautiful as she wanted it to be. Christian Science became her only refuge against migraine headaches and despair. Unfortunately, she also had a strong need to involve me in it, which I was fighting tooth and nail. My only refuge was to bury myself in a book the moment I entered the apartment. In the year 1925 I read everything Dickens ever wrote, one book after another taken in chronological order from a shelf in the public library. Nevertheless the guilt and frustration piled up, finding an outlet only at school and at the camp I attended for two months in the summers. There I found another woman to take over where my science teacher left off.

Dear "Mrs. Matt." I can see her now—wisps of blond hair shaken loose from a drooping bun at the back of her neck, pad and pencil in hand and a rather harassed look on her face, sprinting around the camp trying to solve all its problems. An English teacher in a Boston private school during the winters, she was an assistant administrator at the camp in summer and mother of two little girls—a very human woman, totally without guile or pretentiousness, who felt warmly toward young girls and enjoyed seeing them develop. I was drawn to her by her forthright approach and abhorrence of sentimentality along with a kind of pure, naive idealism which made it nearly impossible for her to believe any girl was really bad unless she was a sneak or a cheat. By that time, I had begun to think of myself as a very bad child, and she did much to disabuse me of such an idea. Although inordinately admiring of girls she thought of as deft, graceful, and assured, she obviously felt the deepest empathy for those who were troubled and struggling. I fell into both those categories, and she was drawn to me too. She let me feel that I belonged to her family for many years after our camping days were over, and her home remained a refuge to which I could flee whenever things got too tough elsewhere. That was another kind of "psychotherapy" for me, and my gratitude has lasted a lifetime.

That these two parent surrogates saved me from becoming seriously disturbed at a very vulnerable period of my life I am certain. I can also thank my mother for the fact that at this stage she did not seem to begrudge my loving them and encouraged me to find my life wherever I could.

Adolescence

BOARDING SCHOOL   A few years ago I attended a dinner party in California given by a friend in honor of her brother, visiting from the East. I knew her as a person prominent in local and national politics; of him I knew nothing at all—certainly nothing to connect him with my own past. When, however, he mentioned being on a fundraising venture for an Eastern girls' boarding school and expressed perplexity at the fact that there was only one class from which he had raised not one thin dime, I turned to him and, without a doubt in my mind, named the school and the class. He was astounded.

I spent my junior and senior years in that school, and I was in that class. I also just happened to be in a group of girls from several classes of that school who were gathered in the smoking room of my college dormitory when the news was brought in that our old school was burning down. With a single voice everyone in the group gave a rousing cheer. It seems that one of the students, probably only slightly angrier at the school than I had been, had set eight fires in three buildings, timed carefully so that all students were in the dining rooms, from which escape was possible.

That boarding school, situated in the beautiful New England countryside, was then and is still considered one of the finest schools in the East. It was a school for daughters of the rich, and I was there only because my maternal grandfather had been persuaded to help with the tuition. Going away to school was common practice among my peers, and although I hated to leave Brearley, I was rather glad to get away from home and not antagonistic to living in the country for a change.

To give credit where credit is due, I never met a nicer bunch of girls anywhere. The only snobbery I encountered was from the riding master, whose face I can still see sneering at my new boots with the contempt he felt toward any boots that were not handmade by a British bootery and well worn on the hunting field. At that moment an image flashed through my mind from much earlier days—a time when Fräulein had forgotten to bring my white pumps to dancing school, forcing me to withstand the scornful glance of a child with long blond finger curls as I appeared on the floor in high-buttoned blacks. Perhaps that is why in the heart of the Depression I spent all my Christmas money on a pair of alligator pumps and would even now rather shiver through a winter without a coat than appear in a pair of cheap shoes. In any case, none of this came from my schoolmates. We wore uniforms, and nobody's clothes were better than anyone else's. I imagine that the fact of our being there at all meant to everyone that we "belonged" and could be judged on our own merits.

Except for the long Christmas and Easter vacations, I cannot think of anything good to say about the school as it was then. Under a self-government system stricter and more puritannical than any I can imagine even in a convent, any infraction of rules was reportable on an honor system as a "sin" at Sunday morning assembly, presided over by prefects in black caps and gowns. "I have done thus and so; otherwise I have done nothing to my knowledge contrary to the laws of the school." One by one we stood up and said it. We were not punished physically, but we might as well have been. It was a "sin" to speak a word in the hall between classes, to whisper in study hall or even say "goodnight" after the last bell. Two "sins" in a week put you on bounds for two weeks, and three or more very likely got you on bounds indefinitely. I was once severely reprimanded for fiddling with my hair in chapel, and when my brother once came along with my parents on a visit, I was told that he would have to sit at a separate table if my roommate joined us for lunch at the local inn.

Educationally, the school had a reputation for high standards, and it is true that almost all of us passed our College Boards with flying colors. The fact is, however, that for two years we did almost nothing except practice for those exams. We would have had to be deaf, dumb, and blind not to have passed. In addition, we certainly learned how to take notes. I can remember an ancient history class in which the teacher started off each session by saying, "At the extreme left margin place a large roman numeral 'I' and write 'The Roman Empire.' Now one inch to the right on the next line write a large capital A, 'The Reign of Pompey,' " etc. We never used a book, we never looked at a picture, we never discussed anything. She lectured, and we took notes. At exam time we memorized them. Anyone who had a nearly photographic memory could simply close her eyes and copy the answers to questions from the notes imprinted on her mind's eye. Large *I*. Large *A*. Small *i*. Small *a*. I got high marks on the College Board (and a few year ago on a cruise to the Greek islands, I finally learned a little bit about Greek history). All this was supposed to prepare us for note-taking at college lectures, and I'm sure it did that. I know my notes were very much in demand for others to copy when they missed a lecture.

During those two years, my anger and rebellion built up to the bursting point. In fact, all the accumulated anger and rebellion for which I had felt so guilty for so many years now had a legitimate focus and could become overt without an accompaniment of guilt. I wouldn't violate the honor code and I couldn't act out my rebellion there, of course, without forfeiting any hope for an occasional reprieve at the Inn with parents of my friends, but I could find little ways to rebel, which strained all my capacity for ingenuity. During the two hours in the afternoon during which we were locked out of the buildings for athletics or walks, rain or shine, I could hide from the weather covered up with coats in a hockey stick box, or read a book by flashlight inside an old culvert. Such doings were not against the rules only because nobody could have imagined anyone doing anything like that. I beat the system, all right, even if I did come out of those hideaways cramped in every limb. I can certainly empathize with young people of today who feel a need to fight a system full of injustice and inequity, even to the point of far greater self-destructiveness than I displayed.

The climax to all this actually came after graduation. At that school, a "Certificate of Completion" was given at graduation ceremonies, to be followed by a diploma after one had passed the College Boards. These exams took place three weeks later, during which time we remained at school to study for them. We were then nearly eighteen years old. However, our emotional maturity having been preserved at the preadolescent level, we seniors decided to be daring and have a midnight picnic on the lawn.

We arranged it as such things have been arranged in every Victorian girls' boarding school story ever written and executed it quite openly just outside the school building on a lovely warm moonlit night in June. Unfortunately, a few unhappy prefects, bewildered by their responsibility for our behavior, decided to try catching us, with the result that, in our pajamas, we fled in great glee all over the countryside and down the main road to town.

You can imagine the giggly excitement with which a group of nearly adult women enjoyed this delicious chase, but I don't think you can imagine what happened the next morning. We were called together in solemn ignominy, and told that what we had done was a heinous crime. We had no honor, we had no decency, and we were a disgrace to the school. For this reason, we would not receive our diplomas.

Most of us had already been admitted to college, and lack of a diploma mattered to only a few, but the only girls who actually graduated from the school that year were a few profects and those who for some reason had gone home early.

That is why no money from the class of 1929 has gone into the alumnae fund for over fifty years, and that is why no money ever will. The brother of my friend, who happened also to be a trustee, was aghast on hearing this story and tried, fifty years too late, to persuade the school to make amends. The administration is adamant to this day, and we still have no diplomas.

Thank the Lord I had been exposed to education somewhere else: almost everything I know today relates in some way to what I had learned at Brearley.

THE NEW YORK SOCIAL SCENE   As I see it today, I never had a true adolescent period. It's as if I sprang from preadolescence into adulthood, missing entirely the stage of gradual awakening to feelings of physical sexuality and tentative striving for intimacy with males. As a matter of act, after the age of eleven, males had almost disappeared from my life except under the most formal and traumatic conditions.

Until that age, contacts with men and boys were pretty normal. I can clearly see the carrotty hair and freckled face of my first love, "Red" McGrew, as he pushed me on the trapeze in the playroom and brought me raspberry candies. With Homer, the farmer's son in Michigan, I gathered eggs in the chicken yard, and later, with my chubby black-haired schoolmate George, I skipped flat stones across the bay in summertime. I received my first kiss at the age of nine during a summer in Santa Barbara, from a "boyfriend" named Honoré, whose family owned a mansion they called a "cabin" right on the beach where we children hung out. We played poker with chips made of squashed bottle tops salvaged from the sand, and placed in the railroad track, swam together, and raced our horses where the sand was wet and hard. There was no strain then—no feeling that boys were an alien species.

During that early period my brother and father were still around, for better or for worse, as were various friends of the family who came for Sunday dinners. During the first three grades at school, boys and girls were in the same class, and in the neighborhood, all ages and sexes played together. But in the fourth grade girls were moved to a separate building, our family moved out of a neighborhood into a downtown apartment, and from then until I finished college, my day-to-day environment consisted almost entirely of women. When we left Chicago, even adult men were no longer in the picture, and my only contact with the opposite sex was through participation in the "tribal rites" of New York Society, to which I belonged only marginally.

The New York social system in which I spent these years had a rigid structure of formal activities, beginning at about age fourteen, which presumably prepared girls for their debutante year. Before then the girl went to one of the two or three "acceptable" dancing schools which, as time went on, held tea dances and occasional evening parties. She then progressed through the Junior, Middle and Senior Holiday dances, along with the Cosmopolitan and Metropolitan, ending with the Junior Assembly as she came out. All these were subscription dances, very exclusive and murder to get into, but those who didn't belong were considered outsiders by those who did and missed out on a great deal of other social activity among their peers as well. Most of the girls with whom I went to school belonged.

My family was not really part of Society in New York, since Mother was a stranger who had few friends in the city and took no part in the life lived by the parents of my friends. She had, in fact, become something of a recluse who didn't do much of anything except care for her household and read religious literature. However, she wanted very badly indeed to have me belong, and I wanted to belong largely because she wanted it so much. She pulled strings. Through connections of my grandparents, I was somehow admitted to exclusive schools, and I was now admitted to this highly structured series of dances along with the daughters and nieces of the real aristocracy of this country. I was recommended by parents of schoolmates who wanted to see me included in their social life, and I passed muster at interviews with the patronesses assigned to assess poise and general presentability. Technically I came to belong, but I knew that I didn't. I don't know how many other people knew it, but I knew it and felt both anxiety and shame. Here again I was neither in nor out and suffered the tortures of the damned to remain acceptable.

When finally admitted into the elite inner circle, each girl was allowed to invite three boys to each of the dances that took place during Christmas and Easter vacations. At these dances, held in the ballroom of the Ritz Carlton Hotel, the stag line massed in the center of the room, and boys straggled out from it to cut in on couples dancing around the perimeter. If a girl was not cut in on frequently enough, she was considered to be stuck, a fate worse than death. I saw boys holding a five-dollar bill behind a girl's back, begging for relief from being stuck too long with any girl. That girl was on the auction block, for sale to the highest bidder.

It would be difficult for anyone not raised under such a system to appreciate the agony occasionally experienced by all but the most popular girls in the group. Even a girl who was usually quite popular faced each dance with a certain amount of trepidation because she could never be quite sure of knowing many of the boys invited to any particular dance. (The mother of one of the most popular girls in the group told my mother that her daughter vomited before every dance.) Coming from all-girl schools, as most of us did, we often had to search far and wide to glean the number of escorts needed for all the dances of the season. and we could suddenly find that at any one of the dances, the boys we could usually count on to keep us going had been invited somewhere else. Therefore, every girl either gave a dinner party beforehand or made sure she had been invited to one, consisting of at least four girls so that, in addition to her own three escorts, she could count on nine others to dance with her at least once. Etiquette demanded that every boy invited to a dinner party must dance at least once with every girl there, but after that the girl was on her own. If a boy liked her, he danced with her often and introduced her to his friends, who might like her too and even give her a "rush" on a particular night. In this way, a girl could become acquainted with quite a few boys and might even have a pretty good time at the dance, but she had to make sure she had enough support to get her started. The dinner party assured it.

I'll never forget the first party I gave. The picture is burned into my mind with acid. I see myself in pink chiffon with pink and silver rosettes on the shoulders, silver shoes, and my usually stringy hair curled after a night of sleeping on hard rubber curlers. Red-headed Barbara in black taffeta with a gardenia corsage. Blonde Alice in blue. Mother had nagged my brother to abandon his customary aloof, uninvolved stance and dig up three boys from his prep school who might be willing to take a chance on escorting somebody's sister, so although I had my three escorts, I had scarcely said more than "Hello" to any of them. I was fourteen years old, and it was my first Junior Holiday party.

Mother had worked frantically for days to make the dinner party nice—had planned all the food, decorated the table beautifully, and hired both a cook and a waitress for the occasion. However, about an hour before the guests were due, she was laid low by one of her migraine headaches and couldn't appear, leaving me to use whatever social skills I had acquired to cope with a totally alien situation.

One of the boys arrived a half hour early and had to be entertained. I can see us now, sitting side by side on the couch trying to make polite conversation. I asked him what courses he was taking at school and he told me; I asked him what teams he was on, and whether they had beaten their rival school. He told me that too, and where he went in the summer, and whether he knew anybody I knew. By the time the others arrived, both of us were sweating so profusely that our clothes were soaked through. Memory mercifully fails me about the rest of the dinner, but I do remember that afterward, when I was trying desperately to think of a graceful way to let them all go to the bathroom before setting off for the dance, I blurted out, "Doesn't somebody want to wash his hands or do *something?*" Everyone laughed, and that broke the ice for the rest of the evening.

Of course, things weren't always that bad. Particularly as we all got a little older, one or another of the boys I met at dances would ask me to go with him to a game, a movie, or some other activity. I learned to tell corny jokes, speak the current lingo, and clown up the Charleston. Sometimes the boys and I had pretty good times together, but after the holidays they returned to their prep schools and I to my all-girl day school or boarding school. I learned how to get along with boys in a structured situation but never had a chance to develop more than a superficial relationship with any of them.

No longer were there casual, natural companionships during the summer. I no longer had a family to mingle naturally with other families which might contain boys near my own age, and my brother almost never brought school friends to the house. Occasionally I corresponded for a while with a boy I had met, but pretty soon there didn't seem to be much more to say. I became preoccupied during the whole school year with trying to line up as many escorts as were needed for the various dances during the next vacation and began to think of boys merely as instruments for getting me through the holidays. This is not my idea of how to help a young girl feel comfortable with members of the opposite sex. The whole thing was a nightmare.

Why did we submit to such a barbarous system? Why do tribesmen in Africa submit to cruel and mutilating puberty rites? The answer to both questions is the same: it is the custom of the culture in which they are being raised. The girls complained to each other and shared their tales of fear and humiliation, but they took the system for granted and wanted to be a part of it. Some who really did belong came through it more or less unscathed and could laugh about it afterward. I laughed with them, but inside I seethed with anger and shame. The frustrations of my home life and my boarding school life were already undermining my self-esteem nearly to the breaking point, and the anguish of the holidays was the last straw. Gradually I withdrew emotionally from the world around me, and by the time I was ready to enter college I was already headed for a depression. That was in the fall of 1929—the year the stock market crashed and that whole world disappeared in a depression on a broader scale.

✳ I think it must be nearly impossible for young women of today to realize how circumscribed our whole group was within the circle of our privileged status. Today, even the most elite schools accept students from many different ethnic groups and offer scholarships to capable children from many walks of life. In my day it was not so. We lived in an extremely narrow segment of upper-middle-class culture and had little knowledge of what went on outside the system under which we grew up. We had almost no contact with contemporaries who attended public or other kinds of private schools, even those whose homes were within a few blocks of our own neighborhoods.

The Brearley School was dedicated to an ideal of broad liberal education for women, yet I believe that in those days it did little to make us aware of how the other half live. It accepted only a few scholarship students, Jewish girls from a handful of wealthy, cultured families, and no Orientals or Negroes at all. The few Jewish girls in the school lived on the East Side of town, and since they were "just like us," we never really thought about their Jewishness or knew what it meant. So far as most of us knew, the Jews lived west of Central Park, where we never went except on visits to the Museum of Natural History or riding on the top of a Fifth Avenue bus enjoying an open-air jaunt across 110th Street and up Riverside Drive. Negroes lived in Harlem, and we thought they were all poor and uneducated except a few entertainers.

We had contact with colored people only as servants who worked down town in menial jobs or as Pullman Porters. (In those days you could still get a porter to carry your bags in railroad stations.) It was still safe for white people to go up to Harlem in evening clothes to hear jazz at the Cotton Club, as I once did myself, but to us the trip was like going to a foreign country. Perhaps I was more ignorant than some of my classmates about the kinds of cultures with which I was surrounded in the most sophisticated and cosmopolitan city in the world, but I doubt that the difference was very great.

Most of us lived within very narrow boundaries, both geographically and culturally. By the time we finished school, a good many of my classmates had been to Europe at least once, but very few had visited the Middle or Far West. As a matter of fact, few ventured outside a rectangle in Manhattan bounded on the east and west by Third and Fifth Avenues on the north and south by 96th Street and Grand Central Station. (The East River area had not yet been gentrified.) Occasionally we went "sightseeing" of shopping in other areas or went to the theater, but that was it. (One of the reasons I was sent to boarding school was that I had begun to sneak over to Broadway in the afternoons with a friend to see movies like *Flesh and the Devil* with Greta Garbo and John Gilbert.

It stayed like that until we went to college. Then, of course, the limits broadened a bit. Bryn Mawr in my day had girls from all over the country, although most of them were from the Eastern Seaboard. Plenty of students came from public and other kinds of private schools, and many of them were Jewish. I can also remember one girl from China, but the only black girl in college during my four years there lived off campus, and few of us knew more about her than her name.

Such ignorance and insularity are no longer possible in the world today. Television, the Civil Rights Movement, and fast airplane travel, among other things, have changed all that. Young people even from the elitist backgrounds I have described no longer feel trapped within a system that they must accept through lack of knowledge about alternatives.

For this they may thank their lucky stars!

3 The World Between, 1929–1939

Before we came to New York, I had been told that my father's business had been destroyed by his enemies and that while he was in the process of establishing another, our income would be somewhat curtailed. However, my mother had made it clear that if we economized carefully, we could still have everything, that was important to us, and this seemed to be true. After three more moves within the next two years, we eventually settled into an apartment on Park Avenue two blocks from my school. It was the cheapest and probably the darkest apartment in the building, but it was a nice building in a good location, and Mother decorated the apartment attractively. I didn't have as many clothes as I had had before, but what I had was of good quality, and, within reason, I could do everything my friends could do. There was nothing to complain about, and I didn't feel deprived. Instead I felt almost constantly anxious.

My problem was a continual awareness of money. Every time I took the Fifth Avenue bus for ten cents rather than the Madison Avenue bus for five cents, I wondered if I shouldn't have saved the nickel. Every time I had to go someplace less than twenty blocks away, I wondered whether I should walk. Not that most people in New York City weren't in the same situation, but to me it was new, and a source of almost unremitting guilt. I could see my mother cheerfully giving up things for herself in order to pay for the skating club that all my friends attended, and there was ceaseless conflict between knowing it was important to her that I fit in and feeling selfish because I really wanted to do what my friends were doing. This didn't stop me from entering into activities, but it was a constant, nagging pressure that reached its climax when I so deeply hated the expensive boarding school for which she had obviously sacrificed a good deal. I could never let her know I wasn't happy there or at the dances she had worked so hard to make available for me, so communication between us, already strained by her incessant talk about Christian Science, ceased except for trivial chitchat about daily events.

Then in the fall of 1929 came the stock market crash, which happened to coincide with the final crash of our family fortunes. I have never known the full story of what happened. I doubt that my father was invested in the stock market at all, knowing his strong views about fools who bought on margin, but I do know that on almost the same day that everyone was talking about the crash a telegram came for Mother saying, "I can do no more for you. Go back to your father."

Mother was stunned into immobility, but not for long. All of a sudden she got up on her hind legs and said: "This isn't going to get us down. I will rent the apartment furnished and make enough income to live in a small place somewhere out of town until your daddy gets back on his feet. I'm sure your grandfather will take care of college for you as well as your brother, so don't you worry about a thing. We'll get by!" Such is the power of faith in God—and a well-to-do father! It happened just that way, and life went on as usual. However, for me it was a turning point. From that moment I knew that as soon as college was over I would have to earn a living and face a brand new world. I think that even as the old one was collapsing I knew the new one would be better, but when I entered college in the fall it was with a sense of desperate urgency.

Bryn Mawr

Bryn Mawr was then, and still is, one of the prettiest campuses in the country—a small paradise of Gothic buildings and flowering shrubs set in the midst of a lush green suburb on Philadelphia's Main Line. Dedicated to quality education for women, it was then the only woman's college to offer a Ph.D., and its standards for its four hundred undergraduates were as high as those for its graduate students and faculty.

In those days, the academic requirements were fairly rigid—a year each of Latin or Greek, science, a modern language, economics or politics, and philosophy or psychology; two years of English, consisting of a freshman course on writing, covering poetry, drama, journalism, criticism, and contemporary essays, and a sophomore survey course in English literature. After sophomore year one picked a major which required a fixed number of units plus a certain number of units in a related minor. A fixed number of hours was required in athletics in the first two years. If there was any time left, one could choose a few electives.

The required subjects could be scattered throughout the four years, but most students tried to polish them off in the first two. There was no escaping any of them, as illustrated by the case of a famous journalist's eccentric daughter who tried to evade athletics by getting an excuse from an indulgent family doctor. Although she was obviously as healthy as a horse, the college accepted this but required that instead she spend a prescribed number of hours sunbathing on the roof of the gym. Refusing to take this seriously, she let the years pass until one day in her senior year when she was informed that without meeting this requirement she would not graduate. Every afternoon of her last semester was spent lying on the roof, rain or shine, and "Sidney the Sunbath Queen" has gone down in college history as testament to the fact that administration meant what it said. Very few students tried to evade the requirements, and in retrospect I am very glad that this was so. Otherwise I probably would never have taken a science, and certainly would not have taken either economics or philosophy. Our horizons were expanded by exposure to fields unknown, and for many of us, the subjects for which we had the least taste at the time were those most memorable in later life.

Dressed in a new tweed suit and with a pair of "gillies" on my feet, I arrived on a hot day at the end of September, ready to tackle the future. I was in a daze, however, and remained so for the entire four years. For me, Bryn Mawr was a wistfully beautiful, relatively secure little ivory tower where I could bury myself in an aura of intellectualism and shut out the horrors of the real world—money problems, family problems, and men. My years in boarding school had destroyed the capacity to take any pleasure in learning. Without the curiosity to search beyond the assigned reading, I got good grades because I studied hard, but most of the time I didn't know what I was doing. In one freshman harmony course, taken to fill in a needed unit, I got an A without ever trying out on the piano the chords I constructed purely according to the rules. I didn't know what they sounded like and didn't care. Methodically I dissected my earthworm, dogfish, and rabbit in first-year biology, having long ago forgotten the excitement of discovery instilled by my teacher at Brearley, and translated the poetry of Terence and Horace as though the words were part of a crossword puzzle, needed to fill in the spaces. English and sociology were still able to strike a spark of enthusiasm, but when I tried to enter a class in French literature conducted in French, I found to my horror that after twelve years of studying French in various schools, I still could not understand the language when spoken rapidly. It became necessary to switch after a month to beginners' German where I could hope to catch up and stay with the rest of the class.

After Fräulein had left our family, when I was five, I had heard no German at all but could remember two words, *"Pantoffel"* and *"Kartoffel,"* meaning bedroom slipper and potato. Why those two and only those two words remained from a nearly forgotten past I don't know; the rest of the language native to my childhood was not only buried but kept pushed away by an active force. When my professor once said, "You have a natural German accent. Why must you pronounce the words like all the other American girls?" I felt ashamed. I felt I was being stubborn and recalcitrant and ornery, but I couldn't tell him because I didn't know. I only knew that it was literally *impossible* for me to pronounce the words correctly except inadvertently. I had to learn German from scratch, took it for the whole four years, and within two years after graduation had forgotten it as completely as I had forgotten it the first time. This despite, or because of, the fact that it had acquired a strong emotional association with the professor and his wife, who were my refuge and salvation throughout my college years.

Many years later, while I was in psychoanalysis, a German word suddenly escaped from repression and led to the emergence of important material. I have now forgotten the exact context, but I remember that in a dream the name "Rasmussen" appeared—a name to which I could dredge up absolutely no associations. Then suddenly it came to me, and I burst out laughing. "It isn't Rasmussen at all—it's *'Heraus müssen'*." ("It must come out.") Soon all the rest of it came out—the material for which I had been struggling. To the best of my knowledge, that was the first and last time any part of my German-speaking past ever erupted from the depths of my unconscious, and to this day most of my nurse's language lies buried among memories of childhood too painful to resurrect.

In 1929, and for a long time thereafter, the word *repression* was not part of my vocabulary. Perhaps I could have learned it in "abnormal psychology," a course I wanted very much to take, but that one was limited to psych majors. Psychology as taught to freshmen meant "experimental" and "behavioral." We learned all about the way monkeys came to fit sticks together in order to reach a banana and how Watson stuck pins in his own babies to test their reactions, but none of this seemed to have any bearing on my own life. As a matter of fact, I found it too irrelevant to encourage me to choose psychology for a major. I'm sure I must have heard of Freud, but nobody in any class I was ever in discussed his ideas in any detail. The notion that one might do or think irrational things because of something that had happened in childhood would have seemed screamingly funny at the time, and the idea that something in my own childhood might make it difficult for me to pronounce German words with the correct accent would have seemed preposterous. However, if the right person had presented Freudian ideas in the right way I might have listened, because I had not totally lost my curiosity to know why things happen as they do. In those days, and even today, what I pay attention to depended a good deal on who was doing the talking. Unfortunately nobody I came in contact with was sending such ideas in my direction, and I didn't know enough to seek them out, even if I had had the energy.

The word "depression" wasn't in my vocabulary either, but I was in one just the same. Throughout my college years, and for many years afterward, a train carrying my depressed self and another carrying the more upbeat me ran on two parallel tracks, both quite visible and well known to me, but alternating in their periods of operation, and each totally out of focus while the other was in play.

On the happy track ran an only slightly more mature version of the preadolescent comic of Brearley days, fortunately now confined to moments of appropriate silliness with my peers—arguing with my roommate about how Humpty Dumpty managed to keep his pants on, or knitting a sweater on roller skates in the middle of Montgomery Pike and giggling at the amused stares of passers-by. The well-functioning self sang in choruses of Gilbert and Sullivan operettas, sword-danced before Katherine Hepburn as Queen Elizabeth in the Big Mayday extravaganza, and won the diving competition three years in a row. Although not interested in holding office—not really wanting responsibility that might require involvement—I was friendly with most of the college leaders and was appointed by them to visible jobs such as ushering at major college events. I had only a few close friends but was recognized by most of the student body and, I found out much later, was thought of as one of the popular set. It still seems strange that the public image could have differed so markedly from the way I saw myself.

Apparently almost nobody could see on that other track the increasingly withdrawn, gradually regressing young woman who managed to find plausible excuses for avoiding dates and dances and was rapidly losing the capacity to feel anything. That me, increasing desperate for some sense of security, tried to find it back in the nursery of babyhood. Gradually worming my way into the bosom of my German professor's family, I spent most of my college years babysitting, baking Christmas cookies, and playing deck tennis in the afternoons with an updated, intellectualized version of Fräulein and a handsome, aesthetic, and *gemütlich* version of a "good daddy."

Both of these opposing selves were able to get their schoolwork done, regardless of the slight euphoria of one and the apathy of the other. I graduated cum laude as a German literature major with a history minor and later received glowing recommendations from the dean for various jobs. Little did she know that I had no heart for any of it and that my hard-bought opportunity for a really excellent college education had been largely wasted. I emerged from Bryn Mawr a conventional, naive, and inhibited girl, depressed and completely at sea about her place in the world.

Connecticut

Every year when October rolls around, I begin to feel a nagging nostalgia for home. Not the California home where I have been happy for over thirty years—not the Chicago home of my early childhood, or the New York home of my adolescence, but the little Dutch Colonial farmhouse in Connecticut where I lived for a total of less than two years plus a couple of college vacations. I long for the brisk, bright New England autumn weather, the flaming foliage and wild grapes ripening on the fence. I long for early wood fires in a huge stone fireplace, funny little winding stairs, and slanting floors of broad boards marked by the heels of time. Most of all, I long for the feeling of family which was almost but never quite attainable there. I wasn't very happy in that house and couldn't wait to get away, but I had fallen in love for the first time, not with a person but with a place. Almost every year now I return to Bloomfield; my niece and closest old friends still live there and open their homes to me. It is still an area of farmers and a few exurbanites, less changed in fifty years than any other part of the world I know. I feel happy with that countryside in autumn and love the people I visit there, but it is really the old house that draws me back—the symbol of past life, not as it was, but as I wanted it to be.

In the fall of 1929, as I set off for college, Mother rented the Park Avenue apartment and took a small cottage in the then sleepy little backwater town of Orlando, Florida, where she could manage to live on the proceeds. Her father had done enough, she thought, by sending her two children to college. She certainly was not going to ask anyone for anything, convinced as she was that my father's difficulties were only temporary. Two years later, however, it was obvious to everyone except her that things weren't going to change in that department. My father felt that his business had been wrecked by bad publicity from the *Chicago Tribune,* which he was suing for libel. Every penny he could lay his hands on went to support his suit, and he would not have hesitated to "borrow" any money he could get from my mother as well as from any friend who would lend it to him. In the spring of 1931 grandfather, correctly perceiving this as an endless process, set up a small trust for my mother including a farmhouse close to the city where my sister lived with her family. Under that arrangement mother owned nothing her husband could get his hands on and was protected from the fear of poverty. My brother had graduated from Harvard, I had obtained a scholarship for my last two years of college tuition, so Mother was free and determined to be a farmer. Nobody who didn't know her can possibly imagine how funny that was to all of us.

My mother was a cute, rather fluffy little person who had several times been mistaken for the movie actress Billie Burke and often acted like her. The thought of her doing heavy labor of any kind boggled the minds of her children, but we were yet to learn the depths of her determination. She had been raised in the lap of luxury and even when relatively poor in New York had always had a factotum to do most of the housework, but now she was not only going to do the housework, the cooking, and the laundry, but she was going to raise her own vegetables, pick them, can them, and eat them. That she knew nothing about gardening would not deter her.

Mother asked somebody how many tomato plants she might need

in order to put up a supply for the winter, and that somebody, probably as a joke, said "Oh, about a hundred." So she went out and bought a hundred tomato plants and planted them in the garden that the farmer next door had obligingly spaded up. Mother had a way with people like farmers, delivery men, and merchants that made them want to do special little things for her. I can see her now in her picture hat and old white kid gloves poking holes and putting in plants, row after row. When it looked as though the rabbits were going to get most of them, she went down to the ten-cent store and bought a couple of dozen children's pink celluloid pinwheels to plant along the rows. When the wind set them spinning the rabbits spun away too, and pretty soon every farmer in the neighborhood had a vegetable garden full of spinning pinwheels.

Needless to say, Mother's plants flourished. In fact, they flourished so well that by canning time she had literally hundreds of bushels of tomatoes. Mason jars of canned tomatoes filled the cellar. We ate tomatoes at every meal, fixed in every conceivable manner, but still they came. Mother was like the Sorcerer's Apprentice trying to keep up with the tomatoes—filling baskets to take to hospitals, fire stations, and police stations, and finally giving them to anyone who passed by along the road. Eventually she had to give up and the plants went wild. They seeded themselves in the nearby woods, where for years afterward one could find tiny wild tomatoes. It wouldn't surprise me a bit to hear that even now a few could be found in remote corners of the countryside.

I had my own day with wild grapes gathered on long rambles through the fields. I too was going to contribute to the family larder, so I got out a cookbook and read about how to make grape jelly. I didn't realize how many grapes I had, though, until I'd filled not only every jelly glass in the area but every vase and kitchen pot. It was splendid jelly, except for the fact that it didn't gel. In the course of reboiling it with a commercial product to make it set, quite a bit fortunately went down the sink and all over the floor, so we managed to retrieve a couple of pots for cooking, but we ate a lot of grape jelly for a long, long time, and I've seldom eaten any since.

Thus we became rural. My brother was there, trying to write the Great American Novel, and a little later my sister divorced her husband and came with her two small daughters to live in an apartment Mother had had created in the cow barn. If we had all been different people it would have been an adventure, but as it was, we had brought our anxieties with us. Nevertheless, we had a few moments of great enjoyment.

The years 1933 and 1934 were the heart of the Great Depression, and jobs were hard to find, but all of us had other reasons for living at home with Mother rather than trying to support ourselves. In spite of all my education, as a woman of that time I had little hope of finding work without knowing shorthand and typing, so I was in the process of acquiring these skills at a business college in Hartford. My sister was having trouble collecting alimony, and although working as a licensed interior decorator, needed free rent for a time in order to make ends meet for herself and her children. My brother, although none of us realized it at the time, was becoming mentally ill and simply couldn't face the world. The paramount reason for all of us, however, was that Mother obviously adored having her family around her again and gave us the opportunity to rationalize our own reluctances to leave by feeling that she needed us.

During that whole year and a half, it was relatively easy for me to rationalize my own asexual and somewhat asocial existence. Although my sister had been a part of Hartford Society, she didn't know any eligible single men, and neither did the few girls of my age with whom I had time to associate. Most of them had recently been married, and those who were still single assumed that they would probably have to leave town to find suitable husbands. I suppose that even at that time there were thousands of nice young single men in that insurance company city, but few of them passed the barriers of acceptance to the social scene. I once asked my sister why some of the older men didn't bring home a few single men from their businesses to meet their daughters, but she said it "just wasn't done" and that anyway, once I got back into the cultured atmosphere of New York I was more likely to find the kind of men who would appreciate me. Wanting to believe her, I did, and reconciled myself to waiting. I kept busy at my business college, enjoyed my first taste of country living, and became acquainted with my siblings for the first time in my life.

My childhood ambivalence toward my brother had abated after he left for boarding school. During our adolescence I had seen almost nothing of him and knew nothing about his own conflicts and agonies. He had grown up to be a handsome young man who talked a great deal about a girl with whom he was in love. It was not until years later that I realized the love affair was fantasy and that he was, in fact, an almost total loner. Now we began to talk to each other for the first time, although never about anything really personal. He mostly confided his aspirations to be a writer and painter, trying to convince me that creative people have a right to be supported by society. Mostly I just listened to him and confided almost nothing of my own anxieties. I saw him as an artist who was different from other people and defended him against the violent criticisms of my sister, who thought he should get a job. My own conflict between contempt and pity for his unsuccessful struggles intensified this championship of his cause. Neither my sister nor I, of course, thought of *ourselves* as parasites at the time, since *we* were working toward the goal of independence.

I had hardly known my sister before her marriage when I was nine, but from the time Mother and I moved to New York I had spent frequent weekends in her home, envied her an attractive husband and children, and tried to make myself a part of her sophisticated life style. Before her divorce I had not recognized the unhappiness of her marriage, but now I became a dumping ground for her resentment against her husband and his "unreasonable" sexual demands. This did nothing to improve my image of men, although at the time I did not realize that I too feared sexuality.

More than that, I became a repository for my sister's intense anger at our father, whose suit against the *Tribune* was at its height, draining off all his resources and every penny Mother could scrape together to give him. My sister, always given to gross exaggeration of everything, portrayed him as an arch criminal, and although I knew the truth lay somewhere between this extreme any my mother's insistence that he was an innocent victim of evil forces, I didn't know just where that was. I had been assured by a number of well-informed lawyers that my father had indeed been libeled but had no chance of winning a suit against such a power. Along with many other people, I believed the *Tribune* to be a corrupt organization that regularly crushed all opposition, but I also felt that the way my father tended to set up his businesses was, although legal, questionably ethical by my criteria. I was one of a group of children who grew up with ethical standards, instilled at home, school, and church, which bore little relationship to the ways things are done in the marketplace to accumulate wealth. I was torn between shame over my father's activities and admiration for his courage in fighting for his rights against such overwhelming odds. Meanwhile Mother was driving us all crazy with her continuously optimistic prattle, but we loved her and saw how dreadful the situation must be for her.

It seems to me in retrospect that during that period I was in a perpetual state of conscious conflict, to say nothing of what must have been going on beneath the surface. I was anxious a good deal of the time, given to crying for no reason at all whenever I was alone, and eager to get out of the house whenever I could, but I had no clear concept of what was the matter with me and felt guilty for not being happier.

There we were, reunited for the first time in ten years, all loving the country and even quite often laughing together over all kinds of silliness. When my sister re-met a childhood sweetheart, rapidly became engaged, and decided to move to California with my mother and brother, I felt a severe sense of loss. Everyone had been upset all the time, and the whole period had been an ongoing soap opera, but all that suddenly faded away in a vast sense of nostalgia for the good times we had had together. Whenever I think of Bloomfield now it is those good times I remember. All the accompanying conflicts and frustrations just didn't seem to register.

New York

On a fine day in late September 1934, I stood at the window of a large room on the third floor of a New York brownstone row house looking down on East 65th Street. It was an attractive room, freshly painted and well decorated, with reproduction antique furniture, Oriental rugs, and two comfortable couch beds. I thought it the most beautiful room in the world because it was mine! My own place at last—chosen by me and paid for out of my own paycheck. Here I was responsible to nobody but myself. I could stay as long as I wanted to stay and do anything I wanted to do. It was my castle. That might have been the most exciting moment of my life until that time. I was twenty-two years old and starting out for the first time to make a living for myself.

In retrospect it is hard to realize that only a little over ten years had passed since Mother and I had arrived in New York from Chicago. Nowadays the years pass so quickly, in such a steady stream, that one decade can hardly be distinguished from another, but those ten years seemed like a lifetime and were, in fact, a number of lifetimes, marked off sharply by the beginning and end of each academic phase: four years at day school, two years at boarding school, four years at college, one year at business college. Now all that was over. I was in the working world at last and was separated from my family at least physically, if not emotionally.

The year and a half spent with them in Connecticut had been both good and bad for me, but they had taught me—perhaps the most important lesson I have ever had to learn. They taught me that around my family there would always be chaos, inconsistency, and irrationality. I might find them exciting at times, funny, interesting, and even stimulating. There might be a strong temptation to stand by to watch the soap opera unfold around me day after day, but I had come to know that along that path lay disaster, that to be a person in my own right I had to stay away from them all. That was a painful lesson to learn, and I sometimes forgot it for a while, but the knowledge was reinforced every time I visited them. It had already become clear to me that there was a craziness about Mother's religious ruminations and insistence on the intactness of a nonexistent marriage, that my brother was at the very least an alcoholic, and that my sister and her new husband were both completely flaky—charming, irresponsible, and totally unrealistic. It was obvious that their lives would consist of one crisis after another in perpetuity, and that anyone involved with them would be drawn into it. I felt very sad about my need to stay separate because I cared a great deal for them all, but I couldn't have borne being with them for even a year and a half if I had not been able to get away periodically into a more normal atmosphere. I had learned from experience that I had to keep some distance between us at all times in order to avoid getting sucked into a destabilizing whirlpool.

I think there is a good possibility that I would have had a breakdown in those immediately post-college years if it had not been for the support of one good college friend and her family. Mary was also troubled in many ways—a fact that brought us together in a close friendship that lasted many years. She had problems with her parents too, but compared to my family, she and her parents seemed like a picture of normality, and in those days I didn't look far beneath the surface. They had a beautiful home where I was always welcome and seemed to be doing the kinds of things that normal people do. I fled to them time and time again when I needed a respite from what was going on at home. Her parents thought I was witty and funny. They joked with me and teased me and seemed to like having me around. They thought I was bright and attractive, so in their presence I felt like that too and got an ego boost to take home and cherish for at least a little while. Their house was as much home to me as my own and was certainly a lot more fun to be in. I think it saved my sanity at a very vulnerable period.

All through my life friends have been terribly important to me, as they are to most people, particularly those who are not very close to their relatives. In late adolescence, peer relationships and healthy role models outside the family did a lot to shape the course of my development. For all young people from troubled homes, friendships with less disturbed peers and exposure to more normal family interactions may be crucial factors in counteracting upsetting family influences, and it was certainly so for me.

I had always had a best friend as I grew up, beginning with the little girl next door on Deming Place; later, the Presbyterian minister's daughter at school in Chicago, and Olga at the Brearley. But Mary was the first one who had an influence on the course of my life. She made me part of a world I had only longed for from the outside. We shared activities, we shared confidences, and we shared a view of life until circumstances sent us in different directions, to end in very different places.

I have often wondered what it cost her to share her family so completely with me, but at the time she seemed to enjoy my company as I did hers, and it never occurred to me that she might resent my closeness to the parents with whom she herself was having difficult times. If she did, she never let me know, for which I am grateful to this day.

At that time there were a number of other refuges to which I could fly for spiritual restoration when I needed it—my German professor's family in Bryn Mawr, my camp "mother's" family in Cambridge, and other peers with whom I spent occasional weekends. But it was Mary and her family I counted on most. When she married and moved away, shortly after my second arrival in New York, I felt a real sense of loss and deprivation. She was the last of my close college friends to remain available for companionship in a man-free existence, and I couldn't help feeling deserted. All my basic support systems had collapsed at the same time, and I had to start adult life from scratch.

✻ I have no way of knowing whether I could have found myself a job in New York in that Depression autumn of breadlines and apple-sellers on street corners without any support. Some young women did, even without a Bryn Mawr degree and a business college certificate. But I didn't have that kind of self-confidance or any experience with battling adversity or scratching against fierce competition in the marketplace. I came from a group of people who, when they need something, seek out powerful friends to help them get it, and that is what I did when I felt ready for the job market. The one who came to my rescue was a cousin of my mother's who headed a large Wall Street firm. Through his influence I was hired as a lowly stenographer in a giant copper company, where a friend of his was vice-president.

I stayed on that job only until spring, but by the time I left my whole system of values had been overturned, and I was never the same again. Fortunately! I learned at first hand about the lives of people who slave from nine to five six days a week for twenty dollars in the stenographic pools of large corporations, eat fifteen-cent lunches at the Automat, and go home to do the housework in dingy flats of Brooklyn and New Jersey. I made friends with Gertrude, secretary to the office manager, a Mae West Character being kept by a bootlegger. Gertrude came to work in a picture hat with white lace gloves to the elbow. I could hardly wait to get to the office each morning to hear about her latest exploits and felt my life quite dull by comparison. Eleanor, secretary to the divisional manager, was another friend—a woman not much older than I who lived in a tiny, crowded house in South Orange, sole support of a ten-year-old son, an invalid husband, and two aged aunts. I heard all about what it was like to be a working mother with no help from anyone and felt ashamed that my own life was relatively so easy. I also learned about the hierarchical structure of business offices, more rigid than the military, where company officers hardly know the office bosses who are the real power, and where secretaries who lunch with stenographers have crossed over well-defined social lines. Finally, and most importantly, I learned about envy and malice and what it is to be on the receiving end of class prejudice.

Dorothy, head stenographer in charge of the pool, was my immediate boss. It took me a while to realize that she had it in for me. In my ignorance, I couldn't understand why it was that the harder I worked to do things the way she wanted, the madder she got. I was so glad to have a job at all, and so anxious to make good at it, that I just tried to ignore her animosity. It wasn't until Gertrude and Eleanor began pitching into her that I saw myself as the focus of an impending office war.

I learned then that Dorothy had originally been hired as secretary to the man through whom I had gotten my job but had been demoted to the stenographic ranks. It became clear that she saw me as being groomed for the job she had lost and, in rage and humiliation, was doing everything in her power to keep it from happening. While I had remained totally unaware, Eleanor and Gertrude had watched her venom pour out and, like mother hens, flew to the rescue of a chick in the claws of a hawk. In a way it was just like the movies—garish Gertrude with heart of gold, champion of the poor little rich girl who had somehow strayed into their midst, and Eleanor, the mother, taking yet another helpless victim under the already overcrowded shelter of her wing.

When I finally managed to recognize what was happening, I was thrown into confusion. It had never occurred to me that people might resent my getting a job through the influence of an officer when a lot of their friends were probably standing in breadlines. The idea that anyone could envy me was too ludicrous to consider. Me! Sweating all day every day behind the yard-long carriage of an oversized typewriter, typing columns of figures with greasy purple ditto-ribbon that stained my hands and blouses. That was before the days of Xerox. Suddenly, in that office, I learned what life is really like for people trying to survive at low-level jobs, and I learned to sympathize with someone I hated. I hated Dorothy for making my life miserable and for showing me up in my smug naiveté. But I could see how she felt, and I hated myself for hating her. It was early life with my brother all over again. The most powerful lesson I learned in that office was to recognize what a narrow world I had lived in and what a terrible snob I had been and probably still was. Before that year was over, stereotypes had started breaking up in my head with a terrible clash, and the headache I got from the breakup was no small one.

✳ I have often wondered how well I could have managed to make the transition between two incongruous ways of life if I had not been thrown by accident into a group of young men and women who were all in more or less the same situation as I. An acquaintance of mine, who knew that I was looking for a place to live, happened to hear that another acquaintance was in the process of converting her old family brownstone on East 65th Street into a series of reasonably priced one-room furnished apartments for "well recommended" young working people. I managed to meet her approval and suddenly found myself in another sort of "family"—a strangely assorted group welded together by our reduced circumstances.

I had obtained a large front room on the third floor of the walk-up for thirty-five dollars a month, furnished. That was a lot of money in 1934 and took a big chunk from my hundred-dollar monthly paycheck, but it was such a lovely room, in such a nice location, that I was willing to eat fifty-cent dinners and fifteen-cent lunches to make ends meet. I had to share a bathroom with two other girls, and no cooking was allowed, but there was a couple named Olga and Gene who for a small extra charge would do the cleaning and furnish breakfast on a tray to anyone who wanted it. Heaven! What more could one want?

In one of the small back bedrooms on the same floor lived Carolyn— a gentle, soft-spoken, rather ascetic young Catholic woman in her thirties, who had lived most of her life in Paris until impoverished by the stock market crash. She now worked for fifteen dollars a week as a saleswoman for the Steuben Glass Company in a deeply carpeted showcase on Fifth Avenue and had a great many connections in New York Society. I had never met anyone quite like Carolyn and watched with some awe as she drifted like a pale ghost between her tiny room, her church, and the Metropolitan Opera House, where she went by subway in full evening regalia to a box lent by a friend who was a patroness.

She seemed to move through a kind of dream world where intimacy with mortal beings had no place, but we all tended to confide our troubles to her even without reciprocation, and when our lives became complicated she prayed for us and burnt candles she could ill afford. We loved her from afar and came to consider her the hub of the wheel.

If Carolyn was a new experience for me, Shelley was even more so. She had come for a winter in New York from Hollywood—pink and white and ostensibly innocent, with a slight lisp and a little ribbon in her red-gold hair. In no time flat, she was having an affair with George in the big front room on the floor below mine, a fact that no amount of sound-proofing could disguise. George was an older man in his forties who had been wounded in the war and worked as representative of a travel agency. Into his room flocked a stream of "clients," mostly attractive women, and there was never a dull moment around him. Shelley was soon passed along to John in the basement apartment, the soulful, alcoholic son of a formerly very rich and now very poor father. John drifted from one odd job to another in companies owned by his father's former business associates before commiting suicide. Shelley didn't last very long with him either and quite soon left "33" altogether. Andrea, who followed her in the little back room, was the niece of a famous art critic, a beautiful, dynamic, neurotic girl torn between love for her Jewish relatives and the anti-Semitism of her New England WASP relatives on the other side of the family. She was given to having hysterics and was always in a crisis with one boyfriend or another but was full of humor and fascinating tales of her amorous adventures. She was my greatest friend during the few months of her residence.

When Joy came, she stayed. Joy's father had founded a brewery in Philadelphia and married into one of the richest, most conservative families in New York. Both her parents were gone, along with their fortunes, but her maternal uncle still ran a large company on Wall Street where Joy worked for twenty dollars a week as receptionist. She was a big girl in every way—tall, big-breasted, and big-hearted, forthright and amusing. Taking after her hearty, robust father, she nevertheless managed with wry humor to blend into the background of her more reserved maternal relatives, who often entertained her in solemn splendor, and she had a rare ability to accept people as they were, without qualifications. She gave generously of herself to anyone who needed her and was a buddy to everyone, male or female. Men often took advantage of Joy's easygoing, loving temperament, but she never held a grudge and drifted through life until she finally drifted into marriage.

Others came and went at "33" over the years, but Carolyn, Joy, and I were stable tenants of the third floor. I left after two years, but they remained and supplied a home to which I could always come at will for at least five years thereafter. Both of them eventually married, and I left New York, but those were years of great companionship between us and everyone else who spent some time in that house. We lived our separate lives, according to the unwritten rule that dates with men took precedence over anything we might have planned to do together, but when we had nothing else to do, we ate together, went to the movies together, and saved each other from the horrible isolation of lone women in a big city.

The parties we had in those little rooms, sometimes with twenty or more people, sitting on beds, bureaus, and floors, drinking cheap red wine with bread and cheese, were a lot more fun than many far grander parties I have attended in the fifty years since. We shared our anxieties as well as our good times. I had plenty of anxieties and moments of deep depression. In spite of all the people I was meeting through my new friends, none of them was a man I wanted to marry, and marriage at that time was my only goal. However, we were all in more or less the same boat, and it made a lot of difference to see that other women had similar problems. Perhaps that wasn't all to the good, because it may have prevented me from seeing earlier that forces other than circumstance were interfering with my ability to form lasting relationships with men. But it saved my self-esteem from complete annihilation and helped me bridge the gap between the kind of life I had known and the kind of life led by most of my contemporaries.

Of all the memories of "33" one clear picture often springs to mind as representative of the changes in my feeling about myself acquired during those years of struggle and uncertainty. On a warm morning in May, I am making toast on the window seat of an open window where gentle breezes cooled the trapped third-floor air. We weren't supposed to cook in that house, but everyone had at least an electric coffee pot and toaster, and we thought nothing of bending the rules to that extent. On this particular morning the breeze blew a gauze curtain into the toaster, and in far less time than it takes to tell it, the whole window frame was on fire—fire racing up the curtains, fire licking the ceiling, and fire beginning to crackle along the molding. In a moment the whole room could have been in flames, but it never got that far because I put that fire out. This time I needed no mother to rush in and save me. I was as cool as a cucumber throughout that whole terrible moment, just as I had been taught to be in every fire drill in every institution I had ever attended. I pulled down the curtains with my bare hands and beat out the flames with a pillow; I shut the window, pulled the blankets off the bed, and stifled the flames along walls and moldings. I worked at it until the fire was completely out, and when the danger was over I collapsed on the floor, as paralyzed as though I had been given curare. I couldn't move a single muscle, and when Carolyn came out of the bathroom a few minutes later she thought I was dead. I wasn't even badly burned, however, and within ten minutes had recovered sufficiently to call the landlady, who only said rather sadly, "Now you see why I didn't want you to cook."

That fire was a terrible shock to me, but it told me something I needed to know. It told me that in a crisis requiring action I would *act*—on automatic pilot, perhaps, but I would take the steps necessary to save the situation. If I had to collapse, I would collapse afterward. That is a very good thing to know about oneself. There have been other crises in my life since then, and it has turned out that way every time. I realized then that in spite of my depression and sometimes despair, there was within the core of me a desire to protect myself and to live. I knew that if a situation could be handled, I would handle it before giving way to panic, and I think I have never been really afraid of an emergency since that time.

✳ After nine months at the copper company I was fed up with purple ditto ribbons and crowded subway rides to Wall Street. I had managed to survive Dorothy, but somehow there didn't seem to be any place a woman could go in that company other than to become secretary to an officer after about five years of working up in the ranks. Feeling confident enough by that time to take some risks, I began to look for another job during my lunch hours. I had learned the lesson about not using pull, and the going was still not that easy with millions of people still unemployed, but, with some experience behind me, I eventually found work in a Forty-second Street advertising office. There my college background made available an opportunity to try writing thirty-second radio commercial spots for Mrs. Wagner's Home Made Pies on a program called "Life on the Red Horse Ranch," and I was off to a career as a copywriter.

At first what I had learned at Bryn Mawr proved nothing but a handicap. Every script I submitted came back covered with blue pencil markings: "This is not a radio word." "Try to remember that your audience has a mental age of twelve years." "This is too subtle." "Nobody will understand the reference." Reduced eventually to talking about "crispy, crunchy crust" and "cherries nestling in their own sweet juice," I began to do splendidly, but in direct proportion to the client's increasing pleasure in these toothsome descriptions, my disgust for the whole project grew until I couldn't take it any more. Everybody warned me that quitting two jobs in two years wouldn't look good to future employers, but at that point I really didn't care. Anything would be better than a career of writing about the succulence of grocery-store pies, and I was beginning to realize that all the routes I had taken led to places I didn't want to be. I had made a living for two years and was having fun living in New York on my own, but it wasn't good enough. I wasn't going anywhere in my work, and I wasn't meeting the kind of men I wanted to marry.

In those days, at the age of twenty-four an unattached female was no longer known as an "old maid," but nevertheless her friends were beginning to criticize her inability to "settle down" and to pity her a little for her failure to attract a suitable mate. This was before the period when such a woman was automatically suspected of being a lesbian—that subject was still as much in the closet as anyone who actually was a lesbian—but more and more, life in that age group revolved around the activities of couples, and a single girl was included in their social life only if a single man—almost any single man—could be dug up to be her partner.

All my school and college friends were married by that time, and in spite of my companions in the rooming house, I was beginning to feel increasingly isolated and out of step. I was obviously wasting what little time remained before the onset of old age and needed to do something drastic about it. Finally, spurred by an invitation by some friends who were driving to California for the summer, I threw all caution to the winds, gave up my job, and with a few hundred dollars of savings in my pocket, decided for the second time to leave New York forever.

California

To someone fresh from the green of New England summer, the Southern California countryside can look very bleak in August. Even in the days before smog, it was something one had to get used to—treeless golden brown hills broken only by the sharp outlines of palm trees and cacti, nothing in the verdure at all soft or muted by shading. In the glare of unrelenting sun, everything looked dry, dusty, and shimmery as Grandmother and I drove toward the coast, away from the horror of Los Angeles. To me the landscape appeared as joyless as I felt.

Sitting together in the stuffy back of her ten-year-old, highly polished

Packard, glassed off from the grim-faced, bored chauffeur, we were en route for Laguna Beach, where my sister and her husband lived in a totally chaotic household of his and her assorted children, trying, without any previous journalistic experience, to run a local newspaper. In those days, one could buy property in a town like that for a pittance, and Mother had recently bought a small cottage to give my brother a more auspicious atmosphere in which to write than he had found with her in Los Angeles. She assumed he would be happy to share it with me for as long as I liked, and although I had no illusions about how happy he would be, I thought it fair enough for me to use one of the bedrooms at least until I could decide what to do with myself. Grandmother's house in town, where she and Mother how lived quietly together, was comfortable and pleasant enough for a brief visit but was certainly not a place I wanted to be for very long, especially since it was quite obvious that any intrusion would disturb their placid routine. In my discouragement over living in New York, I had for the moment forgotten my own wise decision to stay out of the range of my siblings' lives and even considered that I might enjoy living in a town by the seaside myself. That, of course, was before I knew Laguna.

On that particular day, Grandmother was making her first excursion to visit all her great-grandchildren. She was approaching ninety but still alert and interested in seeing a world so different from the one in which she grew up. She didn't leave home very often and showed a certain eagerness as we neared the town, opening a window to let in the tang of eucalyptus and lantana now spicing the cooler sea air. My spirits lifted momentarily too, and we both took a curious look at the place that might be my new home.

We were entering the main street, which runs horizontally through the town—to the left, a row of small shops and cafés advertising "Foot-long Dogs" and "Giant Malts," to the right a rather posh-looking white hotel with multiple small balconies overlooking a wide public beach. Up from the beach straggled a crowd of bathers in dark sunglasses, carrying string bags full of suntan oil and other paraphenalia of the seaside. At the head of the crowd was a woman in a two-piece pink rubber bathing suit. She was undoubtedly the fattest woman I had ever seen outside of a sideshow, and the bathing suit was all but transparent except for a slightly thicker patch of rubber covering the pubic region. The general effect was one of nudity—mountainous, undisguised nudity calmly trotting down the main street of town with nobody paying the slightest bit of attention.

Grandmother viewed it all with interest. Then suddenly a rather puzzled expression came over her face. Resting her hand gently on my knee, she turned and said curiously, "I don't want to seem old-fashioned, my dear, but do tell me—do young people of today consider that kind of a costume attractive?" Grandmother was taking this in stride as just another quirk of the ever-changing fashions. My own mouth had fallen open so wide that I'm sure my chin rested on my clavicle.

The only beach I had known well in recent years belonged to a private club in New Jersey where women had been liberated from long black bathing stockings for only a few short years and still wore bathing suits with little skirts. Somehow I recognized this woman as an omen of the surprises awaiting me. Whatever culture shock I had experienced working in the stenographic pool of a New York copper company paled in my first impression of Laguna. Nothing I had ever read or even heard of had prepared me for the kind of culture to which I would now presumably have to try to adapt.

Laguna Beach in the 1930s was not an entirely typical Southern California beach town. Although small and sleepy compared to almost any such town today, it was even then considered somewhat Bohemian—a town sharply divided between the well-heeled, ultraconservative retirees living in small enclaves along the beach and hills and a heterogeneous assortment of tradespeople, small-time artists, Hollywood bit-part players, minor movie directors, and a general potpourri of drifters, beachcombers, and refugees from more restrictive environments in towns big and small all over the United States. Sprinkled among them during the summer were also tourists and weekenders from inland areas trying to escape the dry summer heat. To someone who had seen nothing of Southern California except the dignified, rather tomblike atmosphere of her conservative grandparents' pseudo-Tudor mansion on a palm-lined boulevard in Los Angeles, the whole town came to seem like a circus freak show. It was in this town that my siblings had, for some mysterious reason, decided to settle, and its people were those with whom they were thrown by the nature of their work and their temperaments. Their friends and acquaintances were the people whom I would presumably meet and among whom I might possibly decide to live. Getting adjusted to that would take quite a bit of doing.

My mother in her innocence never suspected, and I didn't learn for quite a long time, that my arrival to share my brother's cottage had displaced his mistress (as such live-in companions were called in those days). My brother was then in his early thirties; Tibby was forty-five. She had a shack of her own, shared with her twenty-one-year-old son by another liaison, but had been spending most of her nights with my brother. Under the mistaken impression that he was an eccentric wealthy bachelor, she had managed to get herself pregnant without his knowledge and, until I inadvertently let her in on the actual financial situation in our family, had hoped eventually to marry him. By the time I found out what the situation between them was, they were already involved in plans for an abortion. For the first month, I had thought she was just a fellow artist with whom he occasionally had sex.

On the coast road not far from our cottage was a roadhouse named Mona's where all the artists congregated every afternoon at four. I was immediately included along with my siblings and became a participant observer, welcome to their company and their homes, not really "in" nor "out" of the group. This consisted of Dick, a minor movie director, and his "shiksa" wife, Irene, who lived in a house decorated entirely in white—rugs, walls, furniture, everything. We had to remove our shoes on entering, and I was in constant terror of fear of spilling a drink, but they were both quite entertaining, and I liked them a lot. Then there were Eve and Joe. Eve was a bleached-white blonde from a town somewhere in the Mojavi Desert, who was sleeping not only with Joe but with the husband of Barbara. Joe, a writer, was sleeping not only with Eve but with Harold's wife, Marianne, plus girl from a nearby trailer camp and a sixteen-year-old high school student. Barbara had met her husband while she was on parole to his mother from a jail sentence for shoplifting; her father had recently had a stroke and fallen downstairs, where nobody found him for three days because of a party in progress. Harold, who had been a classics professor in a small New England college before he became a beachcomber, was quietly drinking himself to death. Rodney and Molly were Communists who had met hiding under a barrel during a riot. He, a Yale graduate from a rich family in the East, had given away his entire fortune to the Party and was working as a bartender.

Even the animals I met were eccentric. Casey, a dog of mixed ancestry heavily weighted with fox terrier, was an important part of the group. Every afternoon at four, she trotted into Mona's and mounted a bar stool, where her dish of beer was waiting. Jeff, a large dog vaguely resembling a Labrador, trotted each day at a given hour to the butcher for a package of bones, which Jeff always unwrapped before carrying home. This was because once the butcher had played a trick on him by giving him a package of sticks rubbed with meat, and Jeff was not about to be deceived again.

All these titillating items I managed to pick up at Mona's, where confidences were freely shared with the group every afternoon. I found them all very intriguing but had a hard time keeping straight in my mind just who was sleeping with whom at any particular moment and what they all did the rest of the time.

The only people I met in that town who led less complicated lives were Billy, a lively little Scotswoman happily married to a longshoreman who spent a lot of time in Hawaii. She worked as a waitress in the hotel but was well-educated, sensible, and had a motherly attachment to my brother. The others were a couple named Webb and Durlin who had just started a small pottery works making tableware and comic animal statuettes. Later their work caught the attention of the Disney enterprises and became a huge business, but in those days they had an intimate little firm where I got a part-time job for seven dollars a week painting spots on amimals in glaze. The only other employees were the boy who fired kiln and an eighteen-year-old girl from the Valley, one of twenty-four children in a family of migrant tobacco workers, who had herself picked tobacco from the age of twelve but now preferred painting spots on dogs. We all loved each other, and it was only because of them that I stayed in that town as long as I did. I just wasn't brave enough to try to fit in, and I don't think I could have made it if I had tried.

On my first day in Laguna, I found a somewhat secluded beach near our cottage where almost nobody came except a man with a pet duck on a leash and an Irishman named Pat who arrived each morning with suntan oil and a stopwatch by which he timed the exposure of each body segment. Turning himself as though on a spit, he lay all day on the sands and by the time I knew him had acquired the most even, beautiful tan I have ever seen. We developed a nodding acquaintance but were each devoted to our own enterprises, Pat to his tan and I to swimming in the heavy surf.

I adored the ocean—the huge breakers that could at times be so treacherous, the ever-changing blues of sea and sky. I loved all the out-of-doors in Laguna—the dry hills of brush and cactus, where I some-times rode horseback alone in the afternoon, the eucalyptus, bougain-villea, and plumbago growing in profusion around the houses, the immense stretches of white sand along the bigger beaches. But a twenty-five-year-old woman trying to make a life for herself cannot depend solely on nature to nourish her. Contact with nature had always restored me when my inner turmoil became too oppressive, but even the un-limited opportunity to swim and walk along a wonderful beach can't sustain anyone forever. After about three months of indecision, it was on just such a walk that the startling thought first hit me, "I am going to be a doctor." I think I had finally realized that I was never going to find what I wanted by just drifting from one place to another and that if I didn't get into something meaningful I wouldn't survive.

I have never really known why the decision to prepare for a professional career came out as a wish to be a doctor. Even the best psychoanalysis leaves some questions unanswered, and although I gave that puzzle much thought, I never solved it. Did those months in Laguna give me a feeling at some level that my family were in need of rescue from "sickness"? That had been considered, but it seems far-fetched to me. At that time I knew almost nothing about mental illness and don't believe I thought of their behavior as sick in a medical sense, or even as crazy. In any case, to me becoming a doctor at that time certainly did not mean becoming a psychiatrist. My intent, when I thought a little more about it, was to become a pediatrician. I think it likely that deep down I felt I might never marry. Since my major goal had always been to have children, whom I enjoy, the idea of being a pediatrician might have been my unconscious compensation for failing to be a mother. I will probably never know for certain, but I do know that once the decision to go into medicine came into my awareness, it never left me.

⁂ In retrospect, I think those months in Laguna Beach contributed quite a bit to my development. After the initial shock, I learned to be quite tolerant of the strange people into whose company I was thrown and found many stereotypes in my mind further shattered by coming to know them personally. I came to realize that Eve from the Mojavi, Jane from the tobacco fields, and Barbara, the shoplifter, were sensitive, decent people whereas Harold, the professor of classics, and Ted, the well-educated writer, were shiftless bums. (That is what I called them then. Today I call them sociopaths or character disorders, but it's a difference without a difference.) I learned that people can't be measured by whether they do or don't sleep around and that social class has very little to do with character. Those were things I had needed to be taught. I didn't have it in me to become Bohemian, and I didn't really want to live like that, but the experience wiped the sneer off my face and reinforced what I had first learned in the Brearley science lab: "Get the evidence before you draw conclusions!"

That idea needed a lot of reinforcing later, but life in Laguna certainly gave it a boost.

Determined to go to Berkeley at the beginning of the year to get started on pre-medical requirements, I returned to Los Angeles in November and got a Christmas job selling in the gift department at Bullocks. There I learned more things I had never known before. I learned what it is like to stand on your feet for eight hours a day, trying to be pleasant to difficult customers who just might be "shoppers" hired by the store to test you. I learned about sales quotas, and how girls will nearly kill each other for the bigger sales. In that department, items ranged in price from fifty cents to twenty dollars, and each day one had to sell fifty-seven dollars worth before earning a small commission on every sale thereafter. The salesgirl I knew best had graduated from the University of Nebraska and was qualified as a teacher, but her best offer had been from a small town which offered her sixty dollars a month to teach three grades. She couldn't make it on that with a two-year-old to support, and at Bullocks, with a salary of fifteen dollars weekly, was nearly frantic to make those commissions. So was everyone else. Every time a woman in a mink coat entered that department she was nearly mobbed in the hope that she would buy one of the higher-priced items. At first I found selling very exciting and competed vigorously for sales, but when I began to realize what they meant to most of the other girls, I became too guilty to enjoy it. After a while I got my satisfaction from earning just enough above the quota to insure my being kept on, diverting the big spenders to my friend.

The month I spent selling in that store broadened my education in two major ways, one of which I recognized at the time and the other not until later. That was the period of the NRA, and any work time over eight hours a day had to be compensated as overtime. We had to punch the timeclock at exactly nine o'clock in the morning and exactly five o'clock in the afternoon. However, before we punched in, we had to be ready to go on the floor and sell, which meant having the stock all set up, dusted, and properly displayed. We had to sell right up until five, and then come back from the timeclock to put away the stock, clean up the stockroom, and get ready for the next day. That store got an extra hour out of me each day without extra pay, and in the process it converted a totally unpolitical Republican-by-upbringing into a rather active, committed New Dealer. I had learned that one's politics depend a good deal on where one's priorities lie in regard to the rights of people to a fair deal versus the rights of people to make the highest possible profit, no matter what it does to others. I learned that lesson well.

What I didn't recognize until I later studied psychology was how much I had learned about psychopathology. Before I was through dealing with those customers I had had a sample of just about everything, but one I particularly remember. Whenever I hear about obsessional doubt I immediately picture a long table covered with hundreds of little bowls in the shape of a swan, all stamped from the same mold, all absolutely identical. There I stand with a customer who tries for a half hour to make up her mind which one to buy. "This one has a sweeter expression, don't you think?" ("He *does* have a sweet expression, doesn't he!") "But this one seems to have more character." ("Well, he *does* seem to have character.") "What do you think about this one?" ("Madam, I think he's *just* what you've been looking for. Let me wrap him up for you.") After a while she was quite happy to have the decision taken out of her hands, as I have had cause to remember many times in the course of my practice.

By the time I left Bullocks, my shoe size had increased from six to seven and a half, where it has remained, and I think I grew a little in other ways too.

After the first of the year I moved up to Berkeley, got settled in a little apartment, and enrolled in the university. The tuition and the rent were low, and I had enough money for food. All would have been well except for the fact that the two chemistry courses I needed both came at the same hour. In other words, at that university I couldn't complete my requirements in one year as I had planned. In any case, all the courses I needed had started in the fall.

I think at that moment I was as close to feeling suicidal as I have ever come. I had decided that there was one way to escape the purposelessness of my life, and that way now seemed to be cut off. I couldn't afford to wait around for another two years because my savings were running out.

I could and did get a job on the campus that winter, working in the alumni office, but I was so depressed and lonely that I nearly died. The only thing I looked forward to was Monday night on the radio, where I could listen to the Firestone Hour—hear Margaret Speaks, Gracie Allen, and "Fibber McGee and Molly." Almost every other night I cried myself to sleep in total discouragement, all the more bitter because I couldn't let anyone know. I don't know what would have happened if things had gone on like that, but early in the spring, through one of the alumni I met in the office, I was offered work on a newspaper in Shanghai.

I had never worked on a newspaper and knew nothing about journalism. I had barely enough money for the boat fare, and it looked as though war might break out any minute anyway. All my friends said I was crazy, and I myself was scared to death by the idea of living in a strange land where I knew not a soul. But what did I have to lose? I gave up my job in Berkeley, spent the summer with my mother, and in August set sail for China. That was in 1937, the year the Japanese bombed the *Panay* in Shanghai Harbor.

Adventure

The best thing about that trip was that I fell in love for the first time, or at least thought I did. That was in Ceylon, halfway around the world from where I was headed. Our ship never got to China.

The whole trip was a fantastic adventure, straight out of a story by Somerset Maugham, but to go into details would be beyond the scope of this account. In brief, while we were on the high seas, just a day out of Hawaii, the American ship *Panay* was bombed in Shanghai Harbor, and nobody knew what was going to happen next. All passengers were disembarked in Japan, and there was considerable doubt about whether we could get to China at all or, if so, what the situation would be for American citizens. It might be weeks or even months before anyone could be certain whether it was safe to proceed.

For me this caused an agony of indecision. I had only enough money to live on for a short time without a job, and even if I were to get to Shanghai there might not be a job still available. Communications were poor, and nobody knew anything. One thing I did know, though, and knew absolutely. I was not going back to California! Against my protests, Mother had insisted on buying me a return ticket in case of emergency, but rather than use it I would have preferred to die.

By that time I had learned a lesson I should have learned earlier— that there would always be chaos in the lives of my siblings, that if I was anywhere nearby I would always be drawn into it, and that if I was drawn into it I would inevitably be obliterated. Anywhere would be better than Southern California, and since things couldn't be any worse in the East, I might as well go back to New York. A British couple from the boat decided to visit relatives in Ceylon and said, "Why not come along and stop off on the way home?" I said, "Why not? What have I got to lose?" and the next day cashed in my return ticket for a tourist class ticket around the world to New York. Away we went on the old P & O boat *Rawalpindi,* into the biggest event in my life to date.

What I didn't know was that in the Orient, at least on the P & O, tourist class meant steerage. My fellow passengers were forty Indian peasants and sixty Chinese coolies, none of whom knew how to use the plumbing. (If they did know, they didn't bother.) Fortunately for me, first class contained not only my friendly couple but six charming young British army officers with their colonel and his wife, all on furlough from India. Even more fortunately, I was the only young, unattached white woman on the boat. Throughout the whole voyage to Ceylon, they took turns picking me up the moment I left my cabin in the morning, taking me up to first class to use the bathroom, inviting me to hearty tiffins and teas, and both protecting and entertaining me until bedtime. Anytime one of them left me alone for even a moment the steward would try to return me to my place below the salt, but he never succeeded, and the whole trip was one big wonderful whirl of a sort I never had before or since. I learned a great deal about life in colonial India and fell in love with those young officers en masse. Perhaps that is why, when we got to Ceylon, I was ready for Rory.

Rory was a man in his forties, the handsome and dashing owner of a tea plantation in the mountains. He was the third son of an Irish lord—the son who got sent to the colonies in those days because the older brother got the entailed estate—but he spent a lot of his time in England and by chance was scheduled to go back on the same boat I was. We met at the "swimming bath" of a club in Colombo where the British congregated every evening and were instantly attracted to each other.

Rory was a fascinating man, dynamic, egotistical, and witty in a biting, sardonic way that could at times be quite cruel. I found him disquieting and was a little bit afraid of him but was nevertheless irresistibly drawn to him. Nature took its course; on the top deck of the good ship *Mooltan,* sailing in starlight through the Red Sea toward Suez, I finally had the courage to relinquish my all-too-long-defended virginity. At the time I was so overwhelmed by excitement and romance that the actual physical act made little impression on me. I was just glad that it had finally happened!

Everything about that experience was memorable—the boat trip through the Mediterranean, exploring Paris and London together in the autumn. It was a fantasy come true, and I never wanted it to end. We even got to the point of discussing marriage, but the more I saw of Rory, the more I came to to recognize a bitter and rather unpleasant side to his character which, although at first attractive, made me increasingly wary. The ways in which we looked at the world were just too different. To me, the life I had seen in Ceylon was a higher-class, Anglicized version of Laguna Beach, where the British Club replaced

Mona's, but the conversation still revolved around who was sleeping with whom. I didn't know what kind of life I wanted, but I knew it wasn't that.

Before the trip was over, both Rory and I knew it wouldn't work and parted sadly in Southampton. We had had a wonderful shipboard romance, and it did me a world of good, but that was all it was, and I'm glad I recognized it in time. What I didn't recognize until I looked over snapshots from the trip some time later was that he had looked amazingly like my father at the same age. I have come to realize that for a long time my choice of love objects was strongly influenced by an unconscious perception of physical resemblances to earlier figures in my life—resemblances which I could recognize consciously only later, by looking at photographs.

For a good many years thereafter, in spite of lots of dates with men, I was never again so emotionally involved, and assumed I would never love enough to marry.

Returning to New York was a terrible anticlimax, but at least for a while I was no longer depressed. Jay, an old friend from camp, was studying in New York and agreed to share an apartment with me. I got a temporary job teaching fourth grade at Brearley and finally started preparing to take premedical courses. Since I wasn't at all sure of being admitted to medical school, even if I qualified, I spent a somewhat mad year studying premed two days a week at N.Y.U. and studying for an M.A. in history at Columbia two days a week so that I could teach if I was rejected.

It is hard for me to realize now that the time between graduating from college and entering medical school was only a little under seven years. In that time I had led almost that many different lives, each almost totally distinct from every other. I had lived in rural Connecticut, New York City, Los Angeles, Laguna Beach, and Berkeley. I had traveled around the world, fallen in love, and had my first sexual affair. I had worked as a stenographer, a copywriter, a pottery assistant, a salesgirl, a travel agent, and an elementary school teacher. And I had made two lifelong friendships, with girls who really made a difference in my life, Joy and Jay. (Jay lent me the money for my first year at medical school and made me the godmother of her two daughters.) Looking back, it seems almost impossible that I could have packed so many changes into such a short time, but changes had become a way of life to me. None of them quelled my terrible restlessness or permanently wiped out my depressions, but along the way I had had moments of great enjoyment, and the variety of experience was enormously stimulating to my interest in people of all sorts. I have never regretted any of those hectic years, but on the other hand, neither would I want to repeat them.

4 Becoming a Doctor, 1939–1953

Getting into Medical School

Even more mysterious than my wish to go to medical school is the fact that I got in. During the late 1930s it was hard for a woman to get accepted, particularly at schools like Harvard, Yale, Cornell, and Columbia. Harvard took no women at all; the others had strict quotas for women as they did for Jews. Blacks, of course, were seldom even considered. There were even quotas within quotas. No more than one woman was accepted from any one college, no matter how well qualified the second candidate was. With such strict competition, I was crazy even to think about being accepted by one of those schools, but fortunately for me, I didn't know that when I applied.

I did know, of course, that my preparation was anything but ideal. A year of biology ten years ago, courses in chemistry and physics not yet completed, and organic chemistry still to be taken in summer school just before I hoped to enter. I had grave doubts that the bare minimum of prerequisites would be enough anyway and feared that I might be asked to take qualitative and quantitative analysis, which had been required of premed majors at Bryn Mawr. Although I had passed the Medical Aptitude Test, I greatly feared that I might be considered improperly qualified and asked to wait another year or more. However, the idea that I might be refused for any other reason, such as bias against women, never crossed my mind. Nothing in my previous experience had given me any reason to doubt that if a woman was equally qualified, she had the same chance of acceptance as a man. Holding this belief, I arrived for an interview with a member of the admissions committee at Columbia.

The doctor who interviewed me was polite enough but not particularly friendly or reassuring. He spent a moment or two looking through the resumé of my college career. I wasn't too worried about that, but the first shadow of doubt fell upon me when, on hearing me tell what I had been doing for the previous six and a half years, he laughed. He didn't say anything—he just laughed. Then he asked me why I wanted to go into medicine anyway. I said I really didn't know—I just happened to be interested in medicine and wanted to become a doctor. Didn't I want to "help humanity"? No, not particularly. I would be glad to help people, of course, but that really wasn't why I wanted to go into medicine. He laughed again, and I thought, "Oh, my Gosh! He thinks I am clowning!" My heart sank. Then he asked me where else I had applied and my heart sank still further. I answered "No place. This is where I want to go." He laughed again and said, "Don't you know that it's *hard* for a woman to get into medical school?"

At this point I didn't know what to say. I knew, of course, that there weren't very many women doctors, but I had assumed that not many women wanted to be doctors. The few I had met had seemed rather odd to me, and I considered myself distinctly peculiar for having such a wish. It seemed to be evidence of my despair of achieving my goal of marriage and motherhood. Finally I ignored the question. I said I knew I might not be considered very well qualified, but I expected to get at least a B in the courses I was taking and had been told that I might be accepted provisionally. Then he said, "You have a lot of confidence, don't you?" At that I was really speechless and stared at him in total disbelief. I, confident? I, who was simultaneously preparing for two entirely different careers in case I was rejected for medicine? That was *confidence?* He didn't ask me anything more, and I went out of there convinced that I had blown it.

Two days later I got a letter saying that if I passed all my courses with a B or better I had a place in the class of 1943 at Columbia University's College of Physicians and Surgeons (P & S). I had made it! I think that doctor thought I had a lot of nerve and he liked that; he didn't seem to recognize that what I had was not confidence but just plain, old-fashioned abysmal ignorance of the way things work in this world.

As a sequel to this story, I heard years later that in that same year, Bryn Mawr had one of the most brilliant science majors they had ever had, and she had planned to go to P & S. However, practically certain of acceptance by any medical school of her choice, she had not applied early enough. Unhappily for her, I had been given the place that year for a student from Bryn Mawr. I'm told she distinguished herself at Yale while I barely made it to the middle of my class, but that's what the quota system did in 1939 to somebody with true, well-deserved confidence.

I cannot resist one more story about the way women were treated when they tried to apply for medical training in those days. A friend of mine who applied to another prestigious school a few years later was asked by her interviewer, "Why do you suppose, Miss X, that only second-rate women want to go into medicine?" Fortunately she gave the only possible answer: "Well, Dr. Y., I guess for the same reason that only second-rate men do. I guess medicine doesn't attract first-rate brains." She too was accepted.

✳ I wish I could say that I was gloriously happy as I settled down in the huge dormitory that was to be my home for the next four years. I knew that I should have been and felt ashamed that I wasn't, because I had now attained what I had dreamed of on that day at Laguna Beach, seemingly so long ago. I was one of six women and 120 men handpicked for an opportunity to receive professional education at one of the most eminent medical schools in the country. I had been chosen from among many applicants, male and female, for the opportunity to learn an exciting body of knowledge— preparation to heal the sick, pursue high levels of research, or teach others what we were about to learn. I was in line for an interesting and financially rewarding career, with interesting associates. Last but not least, I could carry through life the highly respected title Doctor of Medicine. Why should I not be happy?

In the year and a half since I returned from the Orient, life in the apartment with Jay had been full of fun and easy companionship. Along with my rather frenetic academic life, split between history and science, I had had quite a lot of dates and friendships. I had found a part-time job as librarian on a cruise ship during my vacations, and spent a summer in Europe, and made two three-week trips through the Caribbean, where I met a lot of interesting people. For the first time, "I was living what I thought of as the life of a sophisticated New Yorker, and I was in a mood to enjoy it. Although I had not yet found a man I wanted to marry, I had had a number of opportunities, and it seemed at least possible to think that some day I might. Now all that was over. The East 60s and the West 160s in New York City are separated by far more than a hundred blocks and an hour's bus ride. They are separate ways of life, and I felt that I had again left all my friends in another world—had again moved from one culture to another.

My expectations for the next four years were therefore a little dreary on that long-anticipated day. I was twenty-seven—too old to be accepted as a contemporary participant in student life. I had gone out with male medical students in the past and knew how they felt about "hen medics." They would horse around with their female classmates— be polite for the most part and occasionally even friendly—but they would date the nurses. Not that I wanted to date twenty-one-year-old boys anyway, but I was not quite old enough not to regret the impossibility. I was unattached, uninvolved in any current sexual relationship, and felt totally isolated in a completely strange environment. That environment was a dormitory where the women were segregated from the men, jammed into two cramped corridors on the first two floors of the building, not allowed above the second floor for any reason, and thus cut off from what little casual social activity did take place in the few moments of spare time available to a medical student. I was to be stuck there by the pressure of studies, probably even on most weekends, and was quite convinced that everyone from the world downtown would immediately forget me.

I had known it would be like that, and I had done my best to get where I was. But as I took my first steps into the vast, dark, antispetic-smelling foyer of Bard Hall, I felt as though I was taking the veil—that I was marrying not Christ but a demanding profession that would have to be my whole life forever more. In spite of the fact that this was what I had wanted, prepared for, and won against many odds, depression began to redescend upon me like a cloud, and I started my medical career in a mood that was little short of panic.

Medical School

Of all the mysteries about my medical career, the greatest is not that I wanted to go to medical school or that I was admitted to medical school but that I actually graduated from medical school. Looking back, this seems to me little short of miraculous. When I think about what a vulnerable, confused, disorganized creature I was throughout that whole period, it seems utterly amazing that I could have tolerated four years of constant pressure and anxiety well enough to do any work at all, even the bare minimum necessary to get by. As a matter of fact, I almost didn't.

I suppose medical students of today will say we had it easy—there was so much less to learn forty years ago. It is true that we came before high technology—before CAT scans and electromicroscopes and mammography. The sulfa drugs had just recently come into cautious use, but there were no penicillins, antibiotics, or psychotropic drugs. There have probably been more changes in medicine during the past forty years than in all the years that went before, but that doesn't mean that life is any harder for the student of today. It couldn't be! We had the same twenty-four hours in a day, seven days in a week, and 208 weeks in four years, and we spent that time inundated by the demands of our work just as students do today. Our miscroscopes might have been simpler, but we still looked into them until our eyes felt as though they had been boiled, and we went to bed, if at all, so exhausted that each new day offered a challenge just to get through it.

Schools varied, of course, in the ways and degrees in which pressures were applied. P & S put a high premium on competition and let us know from the first day that before we were through a fourth of the class would have been weeded out. We did, in fact, lose three or four male students within the first couple of weeks, and one of the women died of leukemia before Christmas. Of those who were left, every man—one didn't say man or woman in those days—every man was out to see that he beat the next man. With a very few exceptions, it was only the women who helped each other, because we all felt are were the likeliest to be weeded out no matter whom we beat.

Grades were given out only by the numbers one through five, signifying which fifth of the class we fell into on each test. Even if there was less than a ten-point difference between the top of the class and the bottom, the ignominy of a "4" or "5" carried its full load of anxiety unalleviated by the knowledge that it might just mean an eighty rather than a ninety. There was also something known as the X Factor. Nobody could quite define it, but everyone knew it was there—a certain arbitrariness by which someone's approval rating went up or down without apparent cause. This, we felt, was the most important factor of all, but there was no defense against it, so we just had to live with it. For at least the first three years, everyone in the class suffered some degree of apprehension, although we did our best to hide our anxieties from each other.

"Three" was known as "The Gentlemen's Group"—of course there were no "Ladies" in medical school. A student in Group Three felt relatively safe in taking an occasional night or weekend off from studying to drink beer, go to a movie, or drive to the country in nice weather.

I never aspired to anything higher than "Three" and stayed within it most of the time, although I could rarely enjoy a night off, either because of fatigue or because of the thought that I should be studying. During the whole first year I was afraid I might not get a scholarship for the rest of the time and for the rest of the time, terrified of losing the one I had managed to get. I had become inured to tolerating a certain amount of anxiety and self-doubt throughout most of my life, but during those medical school years I think for the first and probably the last time my ability to think logically and work consistently was really disrupted. On the first anatomy quiz I got a "4" and was practically paralyzed for the rest of the semester.

Memory, of course, tends to retain the most dramatic, and usually the more traumatic, events. Pain has a stronger impact than absence of pain or, for that matter, than happiness, which is less clearly defined. I was interested in many things I learned that first year and derived some pleasure from even such gruesome tasks as dissecting cadavers, but that year primarily evokes powerful visual images.

I can see "Horace," my first cadaver, very clearly as he appeared in a dream at the time, roller skating with me down a steep hill, his arm across my shoulders in a comradely gesture, with muscles, nerves, and arteries all dangling down as they did in the dissection. I can see myself all dressed up on an evening off, when one of my friends from downtown had done the unthinkable by inviting me to dinner at Keen's Chop House. I sit, looking down at a beautiful, thick mutton chop, unable to eat it because there, nestled together, I see the cross-section of an artery, vein, and nerve. My God! I am looking at the sacro-spinalis of a sheep! And then I picture a scene in the lab on the day when we all had to remove the lungs from the chest cavities of our cadavers—lungs black from years of inhaling city soot but so horrifying to everyone that some of the boys had to make a game of it and toss them around as though they were beachballs. The macabre humor of medical students is needed so they can survive the things they have to do. They cannot let themselves remember that "Horace" was once a living, breathing man, spending his days in some pitiful slum and dying without the means to have his body buried. The women couldn't bring themselves to join in the game, but we were trying just as hard as the men not to think about all that.

Those are the images I retain from my anatomy class—those and the permeating smell of formaldehyde, which never left our hands and our hair. I remember those things, and the examination in which we had been explicitly told we were being tested on knowledge of the dissection, whereas four out of five questions dealt with structures in the brain that were outlined in the lab manual but had not yet been dissected. A nice example of the weeding process, which I have had engraved on my own brain.

It was in that same year that I incurred a permanent debt of kidness to all cats, which I hope I have paid off in forty years of devotion to the breed. Most of our physiology course involved experiments on live animals, and although I will spare you the details of what went wrong in what I consider inadequately supervised procedures of various sorts, the whole thing was such a nightmare to an animal lover like myself that I almost left school and have henceforth suffered extreme ambivalence on the subject of vivisection. The strongest image I carried away from that course is of a test in which various parts of cats' brains and nervous systems had been destroyed in order to demonstrate their function. We had to diagnose the site of the lesion by noting the cat's behavior—dropping it from a height to see if its "righting reflexes" were intact, noting peculiarities of gait, and so forth. Of course, a lot of diagnoses were made by noting what part of the cat's anatomy had been shaved, but in any case, it was as disquieting a day as I can remember. What I retain from it now is the horror of it, not the knowledge of the consequences of decortication.

Biochemistry was my favorite subject, even though I often had the lab before I had had a chance to study up on what I was going to try to do there. Good clean chemicals were something I had dealt with before, and at least there was no danger of hurting them. Spilling, maybe. Hurting, no. There the shoe was on the other foot, as I had learned earlier in dealing with a cast-off alcohol lamp from my brothers chemist set and learned again the day I leaned against a sink on which sulphuric acid had been spilled. Anyway, I enjoyed that course although I have had little occasion to use anything I learned from it. The only dramatic event there was when I spent three days laboriously extracting cystine from sheep's wool and found that the crystals I had thrown away were what I was trying to make rather than the supernatant liquid I so proudly presented to my instructor.

That first year was the hardest year of my life to date, but I got through it, and well enough to get the scholarship I so desperately needed. I had lost ten pounds and looked, and acted, like a witch, but a summer working in the office of the British War Relief revived me. It was an active, exciting place, full of interesting people, and I came back to school in the fall feeling that I could probably cope with anything that lay ahead with reasonable equanimity. That was where I miscalculated.

I believe that first- and second-year students in most topnotch medical schools have always suffered, and probably will always suffer, from the preoccupation of the faculty with research and the investigation of complex clinical problems. It is often simply assumed that the students will pick up the basic elements of a subject without having to be taught and that they will profit most from exposure to eminent men (and women?) in various fields. All through our education at P & S we were exposed to just such first-class clinicians and researchers, but unfortunately most of us were not mature enough to pick up the basics on our own and quite often had little idea of what the great men were talking about when they described their research. This became painfully evident at exam time and did nothing to decrease the generalized anxiety. However, one course in the second year was an exception to that rule.

Pathology was the major course of the second year, and one's standing in the school depended heavily on how well one did in that course. It was the one course I can remember that seemed to everyone to be well planned, well organized, and consistently interesting. It was run by a Dr. Von Glahn, lovingly known to generations of students as Uncle

Willy. Uncle Willy had a quality rather rare in that faculty, at least in the eyes of the students: that he liked to teach. He honestly thought it was important for his students to learn his subject and that it was his job to teach it to them. What's more, he seemed to enjoy teaching. I don't know what kind of research he did, if any, but he certainly taught. He was something of a character and had all sorts of little tricks to wake up his students and make them think about what they were doing, but he treated us as though we were people. And when he gave an examination, he tried to find out what we knew rather than what we had failed to search out in the small print of some obscure journal. In other words, Uncle Willy cared about what happened to his students, and as a consequence most of us ended up knowing quite a lot about pathology. I got a "2" in that class, and, what was even more re-markable, Uncle Willy actually smiled at me a couple of times in the course of the year and asked me how I was getting along. It almost bowled me over!

I might insert here parenthetically that all the women were very sparing of their smiles at professors for fear of accusations from the men that they were using their wiles to get good grades. We were very careful about that, and not without good reason. On the other hand, our attempts to be professional and act like one of the boys were apt to generate the label "hard" and "unfeminine," so we couldn't win in that area.

Anyway, I got a "2" in pathology without much smiling, and I think this may have been instrumental in getting me through the second year, because when I hit surgical pathology, which involving doing a lot of surgery on dogs, I almost went to pieces and flunked the course. That could have been the end of my medical career.

Surgical pathology was taught by one of the very few women pro-fessors in that medical school, but no sympathy could be expected from that quarter. She had fought her own way up the ladder in a man's world and was not about to make any allowances for female frailty. Disorganizing anxiety is no excuse for ineptness and, what's more, has no place in a medical school. That's what she implied as she said bluntly,

"You just aren't tough enough for this kind of work, and I advise you to give it up."

I had begun to feel that way myself and might have been tempted to take her advice if I hadn't already put so much into studying medicine. I knew that animal experiments were my very weak point, but here's where my innate stubbornness came to the rescue. I had decided to see it through, and I wasn't going to give up unless I was forced to. For once I had the courage to stand up and say, "I'm going to *get* tough enough; I'm going to make up that course if I can possibly get permission, even if it takes me another year. I'm going to be able to do what I have to do in this field whether I enjoy it or not." We finally compromised on a plan for me to spend the summer working in a rural emergency clinic where I could get practical experience in treating gruesome injuries and learning to tolerate the sight of pain. If she approved the report I would submit at the end of the summer, I could go on with my class; if not, I would drop out.

I had already contracted for a summer job as secretary-companion to a woman writer in Boothbay Harbor, Maine, but when I told her my problem, she agreed to allow me a couple of hours in the mornings to work in the clinic, removing fishhooks from thumbs, opening boils, and dressing wounds and abscesses. By the time I had done that for a while, nothing fazed me any more, and I was allowed to pass on into the clinical years, where I could embark on treating people who might at least hope to obtain relief from my ministrations and had some idea of why things were being done to them. I am very glad I never tried to become a vet!

The clinical part of our training actually started at the end of the second year, with a course in physical diagnosis. Now we could finally pull out the stethoscopes which, when first purchased, had been worn around our necks to the corner pub as symbols of our status as incipient doctors. Now we finally had a chance to be real doctors, actually learning to use these impressive instruments—to tap out the position of heart or lungs and listen to the weird sounds they made. Next year we would be seeing human patients—those strange creatures for whose sakes we had supposedly gone into professional training to begin with, but who had been all but forgotten during the previous two years under a deluge of testtubes and tissue slides. But first we had to practice on our classmates and learn the variations to be found among so-called normal people. One hundred twenty men, divided into sixty pairs and supervised by a number of roving instructors, gathered in a large classroom playing musical chairs as they went the rounds, tapping and thumping each other. Where were the women?

I don't know how they manage such things today, but in 1941 it would have been unthinkable for a group of young women to bare their breasts in the presence of 120 male classmates. Something had to be done about us, however, so we were relegated to a small space in front of the toilet stalls in the women's restroom, where, as female employees of the school drifted in and out, the five of us tapped and thumped each other, and a beet-red instructor occasionally popped in for a fleeting moment to see how we were progressing. On one such occasion, a woman sat trapped in one of the stalls, afraid to come out while the "doctor" was there, and the poor doctor nearly expired of embarrassment while we five female not-yet-doctors collapsed in hilarious laughter. I guess it seemed unimportant for the male students to know something about a normal *female* chest. Anyway, in those days the women would probably have been embarrassed to sit for several hours stripped to the waist while classmates fumbled around with their stethoscopes beneath their breasts. At least some of the men were even shyer than any of the women. I can still see the look on the face of a Mormon classmate when I stumbled into a small room where he sat clothed in nothing but his shorts. It was bad enough for some of them when they finally got to the point of examining patients. Once, in Bellevue Hospital, I heard a tough little babe teasing the young "doctor" who was hesitantly trying to listen to her heart by saying, "I don't usually let a guy get this far till after about three beers," and I remember his face too.

I suppose every medical student has a hundred funny stories about things that happened with patients—things that the general public could never be told without fear of destroying their faith in hospitals.

Most of us tried hard to cause as little pain and distress as possible in doing what we had to do and died a little bit ourselves every time we missed a vein and had to stick a patient again. Most of the students I saw did their best to allow patients to preserve their dignity and treat them with respect. But even so, the system itself allowed things to happen that made me cringe, oversensitive as I was. I still think a lot of them were unnecessary, and are unnecessary as they still happen today.

I have a vivid picture of my first day on medical rounds, when I happened to be the first one to present the laboriously obtained history of a woman who had been admitted the night before. I had spent several hours on that history to be sure it was complete, so I started out with a certain amount of confidence. "This is Mrs. Jones, a white, Irish woman, aged forty, who was admitted in acute abdominal distress. Her husband has been out of work for over a year, and only worked occasionally before then. She has six children, and the worry caused her to drink more heavily than she realized. Preliminary tests indicate that she may have developed cirrhosis of the liver, etc." I really liked Mrs. Jones, and it was easy for me to understand what had driven her to drink.

It took me a while to understand the quizzical looks on the faces of my instructor and classmates, but I found out when the next student presented a similar case. "This is a cirrhosis of the liver with a history of chronic alcoholism," I should have said. It was clear that nobody cared to hear about her family life or why she drank. I soon learned how to give a history, but I was never able to bring myself to call any person "a cirrhosis of the liver" or to stop at least thinking about the kinds of lives my patients led.

Neither could I help being angry when the group stood by a beside and talked about a patient as though he or she was not there. On one such occasion, when a teenage boy's "feminism and retardation" were being discussed, the boy piped up to say, "Well, at least I'm in the right grade at school. I can't be *that* slow." Once, and only once, alas, I had the pleasure of seeing a patient in that situation really rout an insensitive doctor. One of our senior attendings was lecturing the group about a woman's disease and kept pointing out the characteristics of her fingernails, which were typical of a certain condition. The patient kept trying to say something, but he kept haughtily silencing her until the very end of his dissertation. Then, in a condescending manter, he turned to ask what she had wanted to say. The patient spoke quietly and respectfully. "You were talking about my fingernails, doctor, and I was trying to tell you that they were false." With that she peeled one off to show us, and our esteemed professor, flushing to the roots of his hair, fled without a word. I couldn't have been happier.

Most of our professors were fine people as well as fine teachers who cared about their work and treated both patients and students with fairness and respect. However, there were a few sadists among them who horrified us by their callous disregard for the patients' feelings. One dermatologist kept a nineteen-year-old boy standing for two hours, bare below the waist, his pants around his ankles, his arms outstretched, demonstrating a secondary syphilitic rash while the professor lectured on symptoms and signs of syphilis. Whenever the boy tried to lower his arms, the professor would shout, "Get 'em up, boy. You had your fun getting it. This is what comes of it," and the boy would blush in agony. Fortunately none of the students thought it was funny. I can also remember a gynecologist raging at a sixteen-year-old virgin with a vaginal discharge who begged to be examined by "one of the older doctors," making her well aware that "beggars can't be choosers" in a teaching clinic. Most clearly of all, I picture a scene at an oral exam in fractures, where one of the doctors vindictively and with overt intent crucified one of the students before our very eyes.

It was a tense situation anyway. We were all seated around an amphitheater, and in the pit sat five doctors who would determine each student's grade for the entire course by asking him or her one question. Before each doctor was a class list, and they took turns picking a victim more or less at random. The questions varied greatly in difficulty, some from a book that we had all studied carefully, some more unexpected. I was about the tenth student to get a question, which was to read an x-ray and make a diagnosis of the injury. Although I wasn't much on reading x-rays, I managed to get that one right and leaned back in relief. Then suddenly I felt the whole class stiffen. One of the doctors had started to pick a certain student when another doctor leaned over to him and, in a voice that could be heard all over the amphitheater, said, "Leave *that* one for me." Everyone knew how much that doctor hated that student. They had had several run-ins during the course, and although that particular student would never have won a popularity contest among his classmates either, we would all, at that moment, have laid down our lives to save him. Nobody could. He was left dangling to the very last and then, when everyone in the class was sweating, and the student himself was paralyzed, the doctor asked him the easiest question in the book. There wasn't anyone in the class who couldn't have answered that question except that student at that moment. He just sat there with his mouth open, and nothing came out. That was the end of him as far as that course was concerned. Although I believe he graduated in the end, I doubt that he ever became an orthopedist.

Perhaps students need a few such exaggeratedly insensitive people to remind them that patients have feelings as well as bodies that need attention. Awareness of that fact sometimes gets lost in the course of medical training, and we see the results of it all around us, even today.

If at that time I had known anything about the range of activity available in the field of psychiatry, I think I would have know by at least my third year in medical school that I wanted to head in that direction. It was becoming perfectly obvious to me that I was more interested in my patients as people than in their diseases and that my real desire was to understand what makes people tick. I wanted to understand their diseases, but I cared more about how those diseases affected the lives of the people than about understanding intricacies of the disease process itself. Unfortunately, as I have said earlier, the whole field of psychiatry was totally alien to the people with whom I had associated, and the courses we had about it in those days did little to suggest that a knowledge of psychiatry was in any way relevant to the care of ordinary people. Among medical students, as among so many members of the general public, a psychiatrist was apt to be mentioned only as the butt of a joke and was considered to be as crazy as his patients. Some of our experiences in school tended to confirm this.

One of our instructors spent his whole time telling us juicy stories about the perversions of prominent, although nameless, New Yorkers who kept S&M equipment in the basements of their mansions. Another spent most of his time making sick jokes about the behavior of psychotics in a state hospital, although he did demonstrate to us extreme examples of severely disturbed people, wild manics and hebephrenics, immobilized obsessionals and posturing catatonics. We learned how to do a mental status examination and spent a few hours talking to patients in an outpatient clinic, but came away with the impression that psychiatry dealt with "crazy people" who were a breed apart from the rest of humanity.

As a matter of fact, those areas in the field of psychiatry which were later of greatest interest to me were only in the earliest stages of development at the time I was in school and were little known even among psychiatrists themselves. Even if by some wild chance I had done the inconceivable by heading directly into psychiatry from the start, my career would not have been nearly so successful. Given my particular temperament and the way I like to work, each stage had to happen just as it did happen to allow the professional development that was right for me.

I had entered medical school late in terms of college graduation, after a variety of life experience in the marketplace, and entered psychiatry late in terms of medical school graduation, after valuable experience in working with parents and their children at all stages of development. When I finally came to psychiatry, my primary interest was not in theory but in observing people at the grassroots level, moving from direct observation toward theory rather than the other way around. Doing it in that way shaped the whole direction of my thinking. I have never regretted anything that happened to me professionally from the time I entered the working world, hard as some of it seemed while I was going through it. While a lot of it wasn't exactly fun, it seems to me now to have been inevitable.

On my thirtieth birthday, while still in medical school, I received a card from a friend a few years older than I. On that card was the heartening message, "You will never feel worse than you do today," and that message was correct. I never have. I believe that on that day I had reached the absolute nadir in morale and ability to function. From then on it took a lot of steps to get where I wanted to go, and most of them were taken with no idea of where they might eventually lead; but every little step was upward from that point and was an essential stage in my evolution both as a doctor and as a person.

December 7, 1941, fell on a Sunday when I was on call for the medical service at the hospital, doing lab work and histories on every patient admitted during the entire weekend. By the time I returned to Bard Hall in the evening, I was so tired that I almost didn't hear about Pearl Harbor and almost didn't care when I did hear. I had reacted very strongly in 1939 when England entered the war, just after my adventures with all those British officers in the Far East, but by 1941 awareness of the war was lost and out of focus in the pressure of medical studies. I suppose most of the men had thought a good deal about how it might affect their futures if the United States went in, but I think that unless they had boyfriends or family members directly involved, few of the women in medical school realized that their own careers might also be drastically altered. Not many of us in those days thought about the fact that when certain important jobs need to be done, and there are few men around who want them, opportunities for women open up with unprecedented rapidity and bias melts away in the face of necessity.

In order to turn out more doctors for the armed forces, medical school classes were accelerated by eliminating all but minimum vacation time and cutting internship requirements from a year to nine months. Our class was the first to have its graduation pushed forward three months by starting our fourth year in the summer almost immediately after finishing the third. I was put on obsteterics—one of the most exciting times in my life.

During that summer I delivered seventeen babies, each one an astonishing thrill. The reactions of some of the mothers should have been enough to take some of the stars out of my eyes—"Another boy? Oh my God!"—"A beautiful baby girl, you say? Doctor, my husband is going to kill me!"—"A boy? Did you ask the little bastard why he has been jumping around on my bladder for the last three months?"—but somehow nothing could dampen my feeling of delight. I have never been a religious person, but for me the first delivery came close to being a religious experience. As that little head began to appear, then the shoulders, and then a whole living, wriggling child, I felt swept with a sense of the wonder of life. As I held those slippery little feet in my hand, smacked that little bottom, and heard the first cry, I was so overwhelmed with awe and excitement that it took a real act of will not to cry out myself. That scene is imprinted on my mind as few scenes have ever been, and I sometimes dream of it even now. Perhaps that is symbolic of something in me first emerging at that moment— a feeling of coming from darkness into the world as an individual person; but I prefer to think that for the first time in my life at that moment I appreciated what an extraordinary marvel human life really is. It gave me a new feeling for the importance of what I was doing and carried me through the rest of my training with a sense of self-esteem that I had not had since I began.

Pediatrics

BABIES HOSPITAL   It has always been difficult for graduating medical students, male or female, to obtain internships in first-rate teaching hospitals. Those who do get them are apt to have very good academic records or outstanding connections with people of influence either in the hospitals themselves or in the communities where the hospitals are located. For women it has been particularly difficult. In 1943, some such hospitals, like the Peter Bent Brigham in Boston, took no women at all. Others took few women, and usually only those from the tops of their classes. Women were considered to "belong" more on pediatric services, which therefore took a fair proportion of those who were outstanding, but Babies Hospital in New York, a highly specialized research and treatment facility connected with my medical school, did not take an intern of either sex who had not first spent a year at some other hospital. They didn't, that is, until the war created a considerable reduction in the applications of men for pediatric training. At that time, M.D.s with a year of internship behind them were being snapped up by the armed forces, and most of the recent medical graduates were seeking at least nine months of training in areas apt to be more useful in the war when their turn came. For the first time in its history, Babies Hospital in 1943 was taking interns right out of medical school, and one of them turned out to be me.

I had neither an outstanding medical school record nor any particular connections with influence in the hospital, but I had spent a few weeks on pediatrics there as a student, the staff knew I wanted the job, and they decided to take a chance on me, along with three recent graduates from other schools all men who were 4F. When I got there, four of the eleven interns were men, and one, the chief resident, was called into the service after a month. At that point, for the first time in its history, Babies Hospital had a woman as chief resident, and when she decided six months later to accompany her husband to an army camp, another woman was chosen to replace her. We were only three of the many women upgraded and advanced in their careers by "the deed that will live in infamy," and that was only the first of several breaks it created for me. Only in recent years have women in medicine regained some of the opportunities that World War II gave a few of us forty years ago.

In those bygone days, the salary for interns at Babies Hospital, as at most of the other good teaching institutions, consisted of room and board at the hospital plus exactly nothing for incidental expenses. I guess they figured that we wouldn't have time to spend any cash anyway and could probably get along without toothpaste. If we wanted to buy anything, the money had to come from somewhere else. Interns were not supposed to be married, but if they were, their spouses lived elsewhere on other means of support. In other words, in those times, medical school graduates of both sexes provided a large pool of slave labor for many hospitals in the United States (which may be one of the reasons hospital costs in 1943 were considerably less than they are today). Just as slaves in the Old South considered themselves privileged to work for a relatively kind master, we considered ourselves lucky indeed to be chosen for labor in a teaching hospital where the educational advantages compensated for the loss of freedom and creature comforts. As a matter of fact, Babies Hospital offered us perks that few other hospitals offered their interns—every other night off from 5:00 PM until 7:00 AM, and every other weekend. Although most of such free time was used to make up the sleep we lost on alternate nights, we considered it generous, and the fact that except on weekends experienced technicians did the lab work on our patients was a bonus. We really could use a fairly high proportion of our time in learning and caring for our patients rather than doing routine lab work under the pretense that it was educational. On the whole I was satisfied with my lot and started out with high hopes for at least the year to come.

✳ For most of my class, internships had already been set up to start in July in spite of our March graduation, so for three months I moved back into "33," sharing my old room with Joy, who still lived there, and taking a clerical job at the Metropolitan Museum of Art to try to save up enough money for a year without salary. It was easy to slip back into my former pattern of living, and it took no time at all for the medicine I had learned in the past four years to pass from the forefront of my consciousness. By the time I arrived for duty at Babies Hospital, I could scarcely remember ever being a doctor, and if it had not been for one of my fellow interns, I doubt that I would have survived my first night on call.

In those days, the various hospital services were each on a separate floor—ear, nose and throat; surgery; genito-urinary; older children;

toddlers and infants. In addition, interns were responsible for examining all newborn babies at Sloane Hospital, patients in a large outpatient department, and admissions to a floor for private patients of all ages and diagnoses. This last duty was generally hated by interns because there they were merely used as flunkies to carry out routine procedures under orders from private doctors. Everywhere else they had complete responsibility for planning and treating all their own patients, subject only to immediate supervision by chief and assistant chief residents and overall supervision by an excellent staff of attending physicians who made rounds each morning on every floor.

More experienced interns were paired with newcomers on the wards, together covering two floors at a time. Each doctor was responsible for all the patients on alternate nights and weekends, when the partner was off call. All of us worked in the outpatient department each afternoon and followed up on our patients after hospital discharge as well as diagnosing and treating those who had been accepted by the clinic admission staff. Trained technicians did laboratory workups on weekdays, but on weekends we not only had to do blood counts and urinalyses on all children admitted to our floors but also had to obtain and plant blood, throat, and spinal fluid cultures, if indicated, in addition to running infusions, transfusions, and all other treatment procedures, including the planning of infant formulas and diets of children who for some reason could not eat regular hospital meals.

My own service started with a bang. Assigned to the floors for older children and toddlers, I had a Friday in which to get oriented and learn a few of the children's names and diagnoses, a pile of charts to read, some venapunctures to do, and a night to try remembering that I was now a doctor who was supposed to know how to do everything expected of me. Then came the weekend. My partner briefed me on what to expect from her patients, wished me well, and departed. The laboratory technicians cleaned up their pipettes and left. The attendings were already in Long Island, Connecticut, or New Jersey. The quiet of a Saturday afternoon in July descended on the wards, and I was on call. Alone. Responsible for two floors full of sick children, most of whose names I didn't even know. There was nobody between me and utter helplessness except a resident who couldn't be allowed to know my inadequacies or I would be fired before I began. So I thought, anyway. I was on my own. Terribly, terribly on my own!

All afternoon things stayed quiet, and I was beginning to feel well enough to attend a corn-boil in honor of departing interns before things began to happen. How they did begin to happen! The first emergency occurred at about 10:00 PM with the admission of an unconscious child in convulsions. Although I had learned all about convulsions—what they may mean and what they don't necessarily mean—I had never seen a convulsing child and believe me, the first time you see one it is a shock, no matter what you know! it was also a shock to realize that this case would require a blood culture, a spinal fluid culture, and a throat culture—on a Saturday night with no laboratory assistance, while I wasn't sure I even remembered how to do a blood count. Fortunately, while the nurse stood beside me expectantly with all the proper needles and bottles and slides, Alberta came walking down the hall quite by chance and saved my sanity. Alberta was also a new intern, but she had already had a year on the pediatric service of another hospital, and all those lab procedures were pure routine to her. What's more, she was someone to whom I could admit my own feeling of helplessness, and I felt as though I had been fished out of the ocean just before going down for the third time. As we did all that work together, a friendship began that has persisted for forty years.

I got to bed that night at midnight and remained there for about fifteen minutes before two more convulsing children came in—brothers with polio—closely followed by a girl vacillating between insulin shock and diabetic acidosis. It was nearly four o'clock before I finished with them, and I was just about to retire for the second time when a nurse rushed up from the floor below crying for me to come quick. I had never been on that floor and didn't even know that it housed the ear, nose and throat patients, but on arrival I found it didn't really matter who they were. There sat a five-year-old child covered with blood from head to foot from a ruptured tumor of the mandible. I was probably the one person in the hospital who didn't know that this had been expected at any moment and that the child was dying anyway. It was at that moment that I began to appreciate the value of a good nurse. The night supervisor was superb. She was unfazed my glazed stare and, with just the proper degree of deference toward one of superior rank, mentioned that she had already prepared the syringe she knew I would be ordering. All I had to do was inject it, and, thanks to my second-year medical school training in toughness, I managed to do so without fainting. I didn't faint until I got back to my own room. I hadn't disgraced myself, and it might take a few more weeks before anyone would discover what a washout I really was. I felt as though I had been through the war and deserved a Purple Heart. Luckily I didn't realize until later that such a night was by no means unusual and that nobody thought a thing of it. That's the way things go in a children's hospital, and one learns to cope, even if one is oversensitive and plagued by a sense of inadequacy.

I never completely overcame my susceptibility to moments of panic and can still picture a scene on the infant ward where four babies were admitted at the same time, all with temperatures over 105°. There I stood, syringe in hand and frozen by indecision as to which to approach first, until an attending who happened to be there reading charts came up and simply pushed me in the direction of one of them. But such moments became fewer as time went on, and I actually became quite a good intern although I didn't know till later that anyone thought so. What's more, for the first time in my life I really loved my work for its own sake and became totally involved with what I was doing. Every day was exciting and every new problem a challenge. For a while, at least, I gave up all interest in the outside world, and although I still went out with my former friends on my days off, I dedicated myself to acting like a doctor, even though I didn't really believe I was one. Perhaps at least partly for that reason, I was put on the admitting service after only three months.

Admitting was one of the biggest challenges offered by Babies Hospital. Interns on that service were almost solely responsible for deciding which of many applicants would be given the few available beds, and under ordinary circumstances nobody was assigned to that service before acquiring considerable diagnostic experience. Many of the cases referred to Babies were unusual diagnostic or treatment problems suitable for a research hospital, and beds were not to be filled by cases that could be treated routinely at other kinds of facilities even if the applicants were already patients of our outpatient clinic. However, particularly at night, children with high temperatures from ordinary respiratory infections were often brought to the hospital as emergencies; they either had to be admitted, sent home on medication without supervision, or sent on to overcrowded city hospitals providing what our staff considered anything but ideal care. When only a few beds were open, we had to practice a kind of triage—a heavy responsibility and a source of conflict for most of us, particularly when the children we had to send away were already known to us as outpatients. To be on admitting was both dreaded for its painful choices and highly desired for the great educational value of diagnostic experience with all kinds of cases, from the rarest conditions to the most ordinary little red throat. In ordinary times I would never have been assigned there so early in my training, but those were not ordinary times. We had lost two residents, and experienced interns were in short supply. I must have done all right, because I had two long stretches on that service during my two years at the hospital, but my concrete memories include only a few cases that were funny, and a few that were inevitably and traumatically tragic.

One baby was brought into emergency with a potty stuck on his head—treated by breaking the potty in a procedure labeled "Pot's Fracture" (Pott's fracture is a well-known orthopedic diagnosis). Another baby arrived at night having had a blood-red stool and every other sign of bowel intussusception; he almost went to surgery before someone found out he had had beets for dinner. And another baby's mother had mixed his formula with photographer's Hypo instead of the Hi-Pro prescribed by his doctor. One baby's mother blushingly told us as we admitted him that we should know his daddy was a bomber pilot, and the infant would "do his business" only if we said "bombs away."

On the other hand, there was Douglas, the most beautiful two-year-old I've ever seen, playing happily on the examining table. Brought in at 7:00 PM with slightly reddened eardrums and a mild elevation of temperature, sent home on sulfadiazine, and brought back at 11:00 PM dead on arrival from a massive meningeococcal infection that had caused all his small blood vessels to burst. Could I have known at seven that this would happen? Could he have been saved if he had been in the hospital? The answer to both questions is "no," but I have never forgotten Douglas, and I never will.

Almost every day in the admitting room and on the wards we faced delicate judgments and often legal and ethical questions of guilt and responsibility. Mostly we had to solve them for ourselves and live with the consequences.

I once admitted a baby for a routine tonsillectomy after obtaining a permission form signed by a woman who said she was his legal guardian. When, out of all the hundreds of babies admitted for tonsillectomies, that particular one died from unforeseeable complications, we found out that the supposed legal guardian was only a foster mother. Was the hospital open to suit by the real parents? Was I responsible? Should an intern have to check the credentials of every accompanying adult before admitting a child to the hospital? I don't lose sleep over that kind of question, but the hospital was in an uproar for fear of being sued, and it is a wonder that it was not. In today's litigious climate it probably would be, and so would I.

To what lengths may one justifiably go to force necessary treatment upon the child of reluctant parents? Cases raising this controversial question still appear in the headlines today, and one of them was almost my undoing.

Angela was a ten-year-old Italian girl brought to the outpatient clinic with a chief complaint of "pimples." I looked at her chart before I looked at her and was startled to hear at my elbow the deep, harsh voice of a grown man asking me for some kind of lotion. There stood a stocky child with a luxuriant growth of hair on her face, widespread acne, and, on further examination, a large mass in her abdomen. Obviously she had a dangerous masculinizing tumor of the adrenal gland that would soon kill her if it was not removed in short order. Also obviously, she was an extremely important case for research and teaching—the kind of case for which Babies Hospital existed as an educational institution. She had to be admitted, but how was I to get her in? Both she and the parents were disturbed by nothing but her pimples and were simply deaf to all my explanations and arguments about something else that might kill her if she didn't have an operation. At one point, in desperation, I thought I might be able to move the father by saying that she was turning into a boy, but he merely replied, "O.K., we change her name."

Finally, much against their wills, the parents agreed to sign her in for investigation, and the last I heard of Angela she was roaring like a deep-throated bull as they carried her away on a gurney. Three days later she died on the operating table, and the hospital had to furnish police protection for me until the case was settled. Babies Hospital carried malpractice insurance on all its interns, but nobody could cover the cost of the trauma to me, much less to the child and her parents. Nor has anyone ever erased my extreme reluctance ever since about forcing treatment of any kind on someone who doesn't want it.

When precious medicine is in short supply, who gets it, and by what criteria does one make the decision? During the war, penicillin had just been discovered, and only small amounts were available for civilian use. Should I have given some of our very limited supply to a hydrocephalic infant with rudimentary limbs who developed pneumonia? Another form of triage, and who can say which life is more valuable than another? As an intern I often had to play God and was uncomfortably aware of that fact a good deal of the time.

I think the most painful question I ever had to face concerned the extent to which an individual's welfare can be subordinated to the needs of research that may later benefit countless other children. This was a really rough one for me, and in at least one case, the decision nearly cut me in two.

Reggie was a ten-month-old baby with a virulent infection of the knee joint caused by Hemophilus Influenzae, an organism that had been extensively studied by Hattie Alexander, one of our own attending doctors and an outstanding scientist with an international reputation for having developed a serum to counteract it. Previously such infections had been treated by injecting the serum and draining the joint, but at that particular period, the U.S. Government had released a small amount of the newly discovered drug Streptomycin for research. Hattie was chosen to conduct studies on the response of H. Influenzae to the new drug. It was a great honor to her and to the hospital. Everyone connected with the project, including myself, was eager to make it a success. Not only was I interested in the research, but Hattie was a personal friend as well as an admired teacher, and I would have done anything in my power to help her.

Reggie was chosen as one of several patients to receive the new drug, which we all believed would produce better results than the previous method of treatment. However, the research design required blood samples every four hours to determine drug levels in the blood, and he had almost microscopic veins. After a week or so, it became literally impossible for me to get those blood samples without torturing the child unmercifully; finally, after much soul searching and mental anguish, I simply refused to do it more than once a day. I knew that he might be thrown out of the research and that I might be denying him a chance to get experimental treatment that could increase his chances to have a usable knee, but I simply couldn't get blood more than once a day and I wasn't going to try. Since I had been the only one who had been able to get any blood in the first place, that was a very drastic choice, but I felt I had to make it. Fortunately for all of us, Hattie had enough influence with the government officials to get permission for less frequent blood samples, and the day was saved for Reggie. Not for my nervous system, however, in spite of the fact that his knee got well. The anxiety and conflict over that choice took me a long time to resolve.

In the field of psychoanalysis today, there is much controversy over whether a medical degree should be required of candidates for analytic training. I am one of those who believe that it should not be required. Whether a particular person is suitable for analytic training is one thing; whether medical training is a necessary component of that suitability is something else. Many different kinds of circumstances contribute to the development of a person, and it is the person who should be evaluated, not the degree. When I look back over my own experience, I feel that the need to face problems like the ones I have described, under life-and-death circumstances, did a great deal for my development as a person who later became an analyst. Whether it did anything to increase my capacity for thinking analytically I really don't know, but I do know that it has helped to shape many of my social and ethical values.

Throughout the years, I have occasionally told medical colleagues about the kinds of operations on which I acted as first assistant during my four months on the surgical service at Babies, and they blanch at the idea that anyone could have had such opportunities before the fifth year of surgical residency. However, in 1944–45 there were no fifth-year surgical residents available at Babies Hospital, or fourth-year, or third. The intern who happened to be on rotation to the surgical service was usually the only assistant available to hold retractors for Dr. Blakemore and Dr. Humphreys on complicated vascular surgery, which was in the early stages of its development at that period, as well as the usual and unusual intestinal and chest surgery carried out by some of the finest pediatric surgeons in the country. If I had ever had stereotypes in my mind about surgeons as a breed, most of them were dispelled in those months, particularly by Dr. George Humphreys, who later became dean of the Columbia Medical School and has remained one of my idols. He incurred my undying respect and devotion as we worked side by side for endless hours saving the life of a ten-year-old boy named Alvin.

Alvin was admitted after a disastrous operation in another hospital had resulted in numerous fistulae between his intestine and the skin, through which digestive fluids leaked into other tissues and were rapidly eating away his entire abdominal wall. All his major veins were infected and unusable for transfusions, and there seemed to be no doubt that he was a terminal case. Not to everyone, however. Dr. Humphreys took one look at him and said to me, "I can't operate right away. You and I will have to keep him alive for at least two weeks until we get him in better condition. We will have to find a way to get fluids into him, and I'm counting on you to do it." Then he sat down with me and helped plan every detail of that boy's treatment. We worked tirelessly trying to find ways of diverting the digestive fluid before it could do its damage. He worked and I worked, getting into little veins that nobody ever heard of with nutritive fluids, and we did manage to keep Alvin alive.

Dr. Humphreys finally operated, but the next day another fistula appeared, so we had to keep Alvin alive for another two weeks during which the boy, in his delirium, sucked out all his front teeth. Then Dr. Humphreys reoperated, with me holding the retractors for five hours, and after that there were no more fistulae. Nevertheless Dr Humphreys came by every day to consult with me about every detail and to talk with the boy until Alvin, hanging by his knees from the bar over his bed, finally waved us a cheery goodbye. For many years he came by now and then to see Dr. Humphreys, and I have them both to thank for the knowledge that I did play an important part in saving at least one life, and that while in Babies Hospital, I actually was a "real doctor."

In the two years I spent there, the split between my ability to function efficiently with pleasure and my inner sense of inadequacy and dread was wider than ever before. Whenever I wasn't on duty or out of the hospital with friends, I felt a pull to withdraw to my room and play old phonograph records from the 1920s while I sank into a blue funk. However, toward the middle of the first year, my friend Alberta began to break in on that withdrawal, forcing me to talk about my anxieties and gradually disabusing me of the idea that "nice people" keep their troubles to themselves. She simply would not allow me to regress.

Alberta was a very direct, forceful woman of humor and good sense who soon became chief resident, and I believe it was largely through her influence that I eventually became more open and direct myself. We left Babies Hospital together in the summer of 1945, she to enter private practice in Berkeley, California, I to finish my third year of pediatric residency at U.C. Hospital in San Francisco. We shared apartments until both of us married a few years later, and I believe that the companionship we had during those years did almost as much as my later psychoanalysis to free me of emotional burdens from the past that were interfering with my happiness and self-satisfaction.

Introduction to Psychiatry

It was in California that the absence of eligible young men for medical staff positions gave me the breaks that finally turned my professional life in the right direction—that and chance, which is, of course, such an important factor in all our lives. There, in the fall of 1945, I got the opportunity which today is available to any well-qualified woman but which in those days most hospitals gave only reluctantly to any woman, no matter how well qualified. The pediatric service at U.C. Hospital was finally forced into the same situation that Babies had been in, and I happened to be in the right place at the right moment.

The pediatric department had been lucky enough to obtain as chief resident a well-qualified young man who had previously interned at the hospital and then had a year of training at Babies Hospital along with me. However, after three months, the summer fog on Parnassus Hill brought on the asthma that had kept him out of the army in the first place, and he was obliged to leave San Francisco to take a job at Babies. This left the U.C. service in a quandary. Three of the residents, including myself, were potentially eligible to be upgraded to the top position, but all of us had some deficiency. I had seniority, after nine months of internship and fifteen months of assistant residency at Babies, but I had spent the whole summer in the U.C. outpatient clinic and was totally unfamiliar with the procedures and customs on the wards of the hospital. Another woman was familiar with the hospital after interning there, but she had had only a year of training. The other, with a year and a half elsewhere, had some other problem that I have now forgotten. The department finally solved the problem by dividing our nine-month period of service into three parts, one each at the hospital itself, at the Shriners' Hospital for Crippled Children, and at the Children's Service of the Langley Porter Psychiatric Hospital, making and three of us chief resident on each of these services in turn. I was chosen to go first to Langley Porter, and although I knew nothing about child psychiatry, I was delighted, if for no other reason than that the salary for residents there was a princely $160 monthly. The night before starting, I glanced rapidly through Frederick Allen's book *Psychotherapy with Children,* and that was my entire preparation for what would later become my life's work.

The next morning I was introduced to a patient and told to take him to the playroom and start therapy. No indoctrination, no instructions, nothing. I don't know what they thought I knew about what I was supposed to be doing, but in any case they didn't tell me anything more. Gordon and I were on our own together, trying to learn something from each other. If that child is alive today he is a man nearing his fifties, maybe with children or grandchildren of his own; wherever he is, I give him thanks. I just hope I did him as much good as he did me.

Gordon was an eight-year-old boy whose problems centered around incontinence of the bowels and highly anxious, erratic behavior. His mother was manic-depressive, and he didn't get along with his older brother. That was all I knew about his history, and about me he knew nothing at all except that I was his doctor and was supposedly going to try to help him. We got to the playroom, and each of us waited for the other to do something. Finally Gordon took the initiative by knocking all the toys off the table. I, voicing my own feeling, said, "I guess you're pretty scared." He responded by knocking all the toys off the top of the shelf and made for the door. So much for psychotherapy on that occasion. However, when I came by to get him the next day, he trotted off to the playroom without protest.

In the second session, he found some marbles from a Chinese checkers game, set them up in opposing ranks, and said, "The greens and the whites are at war, but the whites can't win. They are too small." He said nothing more during that hour but manipulated the marbles in various ways, finally dropping the whites one by one to the floor. I said nothing at all, because I didn't know what to say.

On the next occasion there was a war between the cowboys and Indians, but the cowboys didn't have a chance because they were out-numbered. Again, before leaving, he poured some marbles on the floor. I still said nothing but was beginning to catch on to the fact that he was saying something and that maybe, if I listened carefully, I might some day understand what it was. My anxiety decreased, and so did his. A few sessions later, the armies were still grossly uneven in strength, but one had the referee on its side, so maybe it had a faint chance. So it went.

Gordon could have written Dr. Allen's book and a lot of others besides. Little by little, he taught me the language of the unconscious, and as he played out his feelings in the presence of a non-hostile witness, the problems began to clear up. His incontinence stopped, he began to relate to other children on the ward, and he began to tolerate his brother on weekend visits home. This change took place over quite a long time, and I don't pretend that our play sessions were the only factors contrib-uting to his improvement, but I think his ability to work out some of his feelings about himself with me had a lot to do with it.

In the last session we had together, Gordon drew a picture on the blackboard. It showed the two unequally sized figures that he custom-arily portrayed, but as he worked at it, the picture kept changing. Over and over he erased the smaller figure, making it taller and taller until finally it towered over the other and practically obliterated it. Then he turned to me, smiled broadly, threw down his chalk, and said, "I'm finished." We walked out of the playroom hand in hand, and as I left him on the ward, I said to myself, "This is it! I'm going to be a psychiatrist." I had not only learned something about Gordon's unconscious conflicts, and about unconscious processes in general, but I had suddenly, and after overwhelmingly, become aware of some of my own. Not long thereafter, I switched my residency from pediatrics to child psychiatry, applied for further training in psychiatry, and decided to go into psychoanalysis myself. It all began with Gordon.

✳ Langley Porter Clinic was part of the state hospital system of California, but it was connected with the University of California Medical School and used as a teaching facility of the U.C. Hospital. There was a large outpatient department and inpatient services with separate wards for children, adult males, and adult females. Residents on any of these services took turns at being on call for the whole hospital at night.

Most people who are not used to being in contact with mentally ill patients probably consider a mental hospital to be a rather eerie place and feel some fear at the idea of encountering "insane" people. I certainly did. My first night on call came rather early in my residency, and although I was by then quite familiar with the childrens' service, I had never been inside any of the locked adult wards and dreaded the day when I would have to enter one. Fortunately on that first night, as the other residents left one by one, I was assured that everything seemed quiet and that I'd probably not be disturbed. When the hospital was finally locked up, with only the night staff inside, I hurried through the silent halls, locked the door of my bedroom, and prepared to settle down with a good book.

I guess the Fates had decreed that my first night on any hospital service would be a trial by fire. Around ten o'clock the phone startled me out of my precarious composure, and I heard the message, "Doctor, come quickly. There has been an accident." My hand was shaking as I put down the phone, my key rattled in the lock of the ward, and as I entered, I was against startled by a voice at my side: "Here is the suture tray, Doctor."

What I saw before me was a cluster of nurses surrounding a large man from whose severely lacerated scalp blood was gushing profusely; spouts of arterial blood were also spurting from both writs. The man had apparently nearly cut the top of his head off, slashed his wrists, and was rapidly bleeding to death. I was supposed to repair this damage with a suture tray? Gasping to the nurse at my side, "Call the surgeons," I walked like a robot toward the patient, wondering what if anything I could do to hold the fort till the surgeons arrived.

At that moment another man, in pajamas and bathrobe, walked forward from the corner of the room and said to me, "Doctor, would you like me to put a pressure bandage on that head for you while we are waiting?" "I certainly would," I said, and all the nurses looked at me as though I had lost my own marbles. This man, I learned later, was a catatonic patient who had stood in the corner for the past year without saying a word or moving a muscle unless forcibly manipulated by others. However, at that moment he was to me someone who at least thought he knew how to put on a pressure bandage, which I had no idea of how to do, so I told the nurses to aid him in any way he requested while I tried to deal with the damaged wrists. By the time the surgeons arrived everything was under control; we wheeled the patient into a little operating room where, as the surgeons inspected, deciding not to remove the pressure bandage, I put in a drip. The helpful patient went back in his corner to resume being catatonic. When it was all over, I myself found a corner of the operating room and fainted dead away, for the last time in my life. Perhaps I never again experienced the traumatic overload of combined shock and responsibility that I encountered during a rooming-house fire and my first nights on call at Babies Hospital and Langley Porter Clinic.

Later that night, I was told that the injured patient had tried to fly out of a closed window under the delusion that he had supernatural powers and that the patient who had put on the bandage was formerly an orthopedic surgeon who, since becoming ill a few years earlier, had never before broken out of his catatonic trance. For weeks afterward, I went to his ward daily to visit with him—to try getting through to him my gratitude for his aid at a moment of crisis, and to demonstrate to him his continuing value to the world as a functioning person. However, he never, by even the flicker of an eyelash, gave any indication that he even heard me, and in the end I had to give up and go back to try communicating with my own patients.

That man's performance on that night unfortunately did him no permanent good so far as I know, but the good it did for me is incalculable. It not only brought me out of a state of shock and helped me to function effectively at a moment of crisis, but it taught me, under the most dramatic and moving of circumstances, to take a new look at "insanity" and to realize that mental illness does not remove the essential humanity of people so afflicted. It sent me into psychiatric training with not only an interest and awareness of unconscious mental processes but with a keen concern and feeling for the severely disturbed as people with strengths that could be utilized to help them get well if only they could be mobilized. Again I had the opportunity to approach learning from a direct experience rather than from theoretical knowledge, and I have been thankful ever since to the man who first showed me that a schizophrenic patient still has within him the qualities and mental capacities of a person. This happened even before I learned that someone who had been very close to me as a person had within him the qualities and mental capacities of a schizophrenic patient.

　　　　　　　　　　　　✻ During the early years after my return to California, my personal life was in a state of almost continual upheaval. I had known, of course, that coming back to within four hundred miles of my family would entail a certain amount of complexity, but nobody could have predicted the volume of Sturm and Drang that began almost immediately and accelerated with increasing speed until I nearly drowned in a whirlpool of emotions, my own and everyone else's. Professionally, those years went along smoothly, with steady progress in capability and success. Personally, my life was a shambles.

After living for short periods in a series of the cramped, unattractive apartments that were all one could find in overcrowded, immediate postwar Berkeley, I discovered through a newspaper ad that a house was for sale in nearby Point Richmond at quite a reasonable price and decided to take a look at it. Point Richmond is a small, rather offbeat community on the shore of the Bay—a semirural island contained within the industrial city of Richmond, which, at that time, was still home for the Kaiser Shipbuilding Industries. Although a number of artists and university professors had managed to find the place, most people had never heard of "The Point," nor had I. However, from the moment I laid eyes on it, Point Richmond became the answer to a dream, and that house became a dream house for which I would have sold my soul. I had to have it, no matter what I would have to do to get it. By that time my grandmother had died, and my mother's trust officer allowed her to loan me the money for a down payment. Loaded with debts and mortgages, I moved in along with Alberta and two cats. We had almost no furniture and almost nothing else to make the place habitable, but there was plenty of room, a beautiful garden, and a big deck looking out to the Bay practically in our front yard. We were as happy as could be until our families and some of our friends decided they now had a free crash pad available, away from the stresses of their own domestic arrangements. From then on, we all but ran a hotel, with her siblings and mine, separately and together, drifting in and out for weeks, sometimes months, at a time, bringing with them all the horrors of their terribly complicated lives. As one crisis-prone individual after another dumped emotional garbage on our heads, our own tensions mounted and mounted. Neither of us had the courage to set limits— engulfed in anger and frustration mingled with compassion and a wish to help, we were both powerless to say "No more!"

Almost at the same time I returned to the West, my father had re-entered my mother's life and managed to embroil her in his always unusual business affairs. Shortly afterward, both were indicted for mail fraud. What they were doing, odd as it was, was perfectly legal, and when it finally came up the case was thrown out of court with a rebuke to the government agency that had brought it; but anxiety about it dragged on for months, with all of us worried to death about what might happen to Mother. My sister was consumed with fury both at our father and her husband, who was carrying on with other women, and she was becoming increasingly alcoholic. She and Alberta hated each other, but I felt so sorry for her that I repeatedly let her come, while Alberta, in turn, could not refuse to let her sister bring her lover and two dogs to rent rooms in our basement. Her teenage brother brought his girlfriends serially to stay for nights and lots of weekends, while my brother-in-law came to plead his case whenever my sister wasn't there. My own brother, who was there so often he practically lived with us, was clearly becoming psychotic, talking incessantly about the New World a-coming in which he would be the Messiah. It took us a while to recognize his condition, but soon it became impossible to avoid seeing what was happening and recognizing that a suicide attempt would be only a matter of time. He refused to get psychiatric help, Mother refused to recognize that we was ill; and there was nothing we could do about it. Anger, anxiety, and suspense were our daily fare. After a while Alberta got married, moved out, and had a baby. I had to adjust to being again without a companion to share my life—and to my envy of her for getting what I myself so desperately wanted. Later, I had to adjust to falling in love myself and starting an affair that might or might not end in marriage. On top of all this, I was accepted as a candidate by the San Francisco Psychoanalytic Institute and started a training analysis with Professor Erik Erikson.

All this reminds me of the story about a woman from a small Russian village who went to see the rabbi, telling him her life was unbearable. She and her husband lived with their parents and six children in a tiny cottage with scarcely room to breathe, but there was no way any of them could move out. The rabbi said, "Have you a goat?" When she said "yes," he advised her to take the goat into the house. The next week she came back saying that now life was *absolutely* unbearable, whereupon he advised her to take in the cow. Next week the chickens. Finally, when she was clearly at the breaking point, he suggested that she take out the chickens. Then the cow. Then the goat. Week by week. By the time all the animals were gone, she felt she had so much room that she went about her business and bothered him no more.

Taking on analysis on top of everything else that was going on in my house was like taking in the chickens, the cow, and the goat. Now, in addition to anxiety over my mother's fate and my sister's and my brother's, I had to face the anxieties produced by wild, frightening dreams, the development of transference feelings, and the gradual release of painful, repressed memories. However, I was determined to do it, and I had found, I firmly believe, one of the few training analysts in the world who would have taken me on under those circumstances. I'm not sure he realized what he was getting into when we began, but he didn't desert me when he found out, and we struggled through three years of it together. It added stress to my life, but it also gave me the support I needed to get through it. Eventually I learned to say "NO!" to my sister and my brother-in-law, and I learned to let my parents lead their own lives without my having to bleed over everything that happened to them. When my brother's suicide finally took place, I was able to bear it without totally collapsing myself. The ability to cope with pressures from my family in itself would have been a good result from analysis, but in addition I gradually got rid of the conflicts that had been standing in the way of my ability to make a close, lasting relationship with a man. A little later I did marry and remained happily married until my husband's death twenty years later. We were never able to have children, but I even learned to cope with that and to become reconciled to settling for two teenage stepsons and step grand- ? p 149 children as they came along. As a matter of fact, that was a very happy solution for me; I had all the fun of participating in the development of a young family without the struggles of trying to combine an active professional life with raising small children. It all worked out in the end, but what a time it was getting to that point!

✻ I believe that the reasonably serene and uninterrupted progress of my professional life, alongside all the turmoil, can only be explained by the fact that my whole personality developed on two parallel tracks right from the beginning. After the age of six weeks, I grew up leading two separate but concomitant lives, with two separate but concomitant families in which I played quite different roles and had quite different feelings about myself.

Among the members of my family, I grew up feeling excluded and less loved. Within that context, a side of me developed that tends always to question my adequacy and sense of belonging. Everything connected with my parents and siblings was fraught with anxiety and ambivalence, keeping me depressed and preoccupied with them and their problems for thirty-five years.

In the relationship to my nurse, however, I felt quite good about myself—a feeling based on the solid foundation of being exclusively loved and considered important. As the adored "only child" of a down-to-earth, rather unimaginative "mother," I belonged to a world that valued me and thus came to look upon myself as both capable and lovable—lovable, that is, to mother figures. Later relationships in school and on the job tended to reinforce that self-image, and I learned to find among playmates and friends at each stage of development one prime companion who, like my nurse, served as an anchor for the feeling of being O.K. Although never entirely sure of myself, I could function well in the world outside my family except for the brief period during medical school when I had no such anchor.

Feelings of depression and despair, which were always perfectly conscious when they occurred, never seriously invaded my ability to work or destroyed my ability to enjoy life, while feelings of self-confidence and security derived from successes in the outside world never were evident in dealings with my family. It took psychoanalysis to pull together the polarized fragments of self-esteem and create a self-image of someone who could both work and love without anxiety. I think, however, that I remain a person who will always have somewhat divided loyalties—between work and personal life, and between various lines of interest within my field of endeavor. Fortunately, this has never created major conflict and has added considerable breadth to my professional life.

5 Emerging into the Field of Psychiatry

The particular period in the 1940s when I completed training at Langley Porter was the ideal time for anyone, male or female, to start a private practice in psychiatry in Berkeley. There was only a small handful of overworked psychiatrists in the whole East Bay area, only one of them female. However, it was not compatible with either my temperament or my pocketbook to start right out boldly by opening an office, and although I needed to make some money fast, it never occurred to me that I could possibly be capable of hanging out a shingle immediately and getting patients. Some months later, when I finally did have the courage to open an office part-time, the available hours were filled within a week, as were all the hours offered by anyone starting at that time, but I certainly hadn't expected it to be like that.

At first I knew only that I had to assure myself of enough steady income to cover my living expenses plus heavy mortgages, and since it had always been my pattern to cope with uncertainty with plenty of alternatives, I signed up for two part-time jobs before even considering anything else. In so doing, I hit upon a great piece of luck—not because there were few men around at the time or because the situation called for a woman, but because I happened to need money at a particular moment and was personally insecure enough to seek part-time work in a health department. Just at the time of my application, the city of Berkeley was in great need of someone with exactly the combination of qualifications I had, and there was no one else around of any sex who had that particular combination.

In 1946, the community psychiatry movement had not yet gained momentum. Mental health planners were still thinking in terms of providing more treatment facilities for disturbed adults and developing child guidance clinics for the treatment of disturbed children. Few people were thinking much about how such disturbances might be prevented. However, there were a few far-sighted professional people in both psychiatry and pediatrics who were beginning to realize that treatment facilities alone would never meet the need for help with emotional problems, if for no other reason than that the vast majority of people in need of such help do not seek it in a psychiatric clinic and are, in fact, afraid to do so. These professionals were thinking that for many such people, help in both preventing and relieving emotional stress might best be offered by personnel of various public agencies, who see many kinds of people in the course of rendering nonpsychiatric services. Public health nurses, nursery school teachers, and teachers at all levels of the public school system night be in a particularly advantageous position to help relieve the anxieties of parents and children before more serious disturbances occurred if they were taught to recognize warning signs and were relieved of their anxieties in dealing with problems through the exercise of their own skills.

Dr. Paul Lemkau in Baltimore had already introduced a program of consultation for public health nurses and was shortly to publish *Mental Hygiene in Public Health* (1949). In New York, Dr. Leona Baumgartner had set up a similar program, and Dr. Gerald Caplan in Boston was developing facilities for training psychiatrists to consult with personnel in various types of community agency. Drs. Milton Senn, Benjamin Spock, and David Levy, to name only a few, were among those who appreciated the important role pediatricians could play in helping parents avoid problems through "healthy" child-rearing practices, and Dr. Julius Levy in Newark, N.J. was training pediatricians in a program of "anticipatory guidance" to aid parents of children attending well-baby clinics. All these programs were just starting and were little known to the majority of professional people in psychiatry, public health, or pediatrics. I myself had never heard of them.

At this particular period, Berkeley had a very active and aggressive Mental Hygiene Association that had been putting great pressure on the city to set up a child guidance clinic within the Health Department. City officials, were leery of the whole idea, feeling that offering direct service was not the function of a health department. Dr. Frank Kelly, the chief health officer, was especially balky at pressure from what he lovingly called "The Plague of Women Voters" and "The Mental Hygiene Assassination." Although a committee of consultants under the auspices of the Commonwealth Fund had been invited by these bodies to evaluate the local situation, he was little inclined to cooperate. He was a stubborn Irishman who didn't like people sticking their noses into his affairs, he didn't trust psychiatrists anyway, and he wasn't about to have any of them mouthing their jargon around his department! It looked as though war would be declared at any moment.

It was just at this moment that I happened to show up on his doorstep asking for a job—any part-time job that would cover my mortgage payments. He asked me what I thought I could contribute to a health department, and I told him I thought my psychiatric training might be usefully combined with my experience in pediatrics by setting up a guidance program for parents in well-baby clinics, centered around discussion of ordinary developmental stages and expectations. I didn't know it then, of course, but I was the answer to Dr. Kelly's prayer! He didn't have to hire a psychiatrist! He could hire a "cute chick" with enough qualifications to shut the mouths of those "Plagues" and "Assassinations," and he could do it before the evaluating committee ever got to Berkeley! Dr. Kelly didn't care much for women doctors, but he was partial to "cute chicks." Clapping me on the shoulder he said, "It's all yours, Baby! Set up what you think is a good mental health program for a health department, and have it operating in a month." And I did.

He gave me a completely free hand, and we became the greatest of friends. If I do say it myself, we set up a splendid program, focused on making various types of public health workers aware of their value in promoting the mental health of their patients, not by teaching the workers to do psychotherapy, but by teaching them how to be more aware of the emotional interactions taking place in the normal use of their own skills. I wrote it all up later in a book called *Mental Health In-service Training* (1968), which was very well reviewed although I don't think anyone paid much attention to it. I still think there should be more programs like it, but unfortunately the community psychiatry movement went in another direction and finally died out.

So far as Frank Kelly was concerned, the important thing was that the evaluating committee loved it and got the "Plague of Women Voters" off his back. The important thing for me was that I got a lot of valuable experience working with different kinds of groups and applying psychoanalytic concepts to many disparate kinds of situations. Better still, I came into close personal contact with leaders in some of the most interesting developments taking place in the field of mental health throughout the country and made a lot of good friends among them.

In the summer of 1948, an institute of Mental Health in Public Health was held in Berkeley under the auspices of the Commonwealth Fund and the California State Department of Mental Health. A distinguished faculty from all over the country—eight psychiatrists, three pediatricians with psychiatric training, including Spock and Milton Senn, and five public health leaders, including Leona Baumgartner— worked intensively for two weeks with a group of California health officers, giving them a view of public health's potential role in human relationships (a description of this project was later published as a book by Ethel L. Ginsburg called *Public Health Is People* [1950]). Dr. Kelly and I both participated. He got a lot of praise from the faculty for being a pioneer in recognizing the importance of mental health in his department and became an enthusiastic convert. I became supporter of the community psychiatry movement for many years, was on the faculty of the short-lived Center for Training in Community Psychiatry in Berkeley under the direction of Dr. Portia Hume, and gave a graduate course on mental health in the University of California School of Public Health. The whole experience was not only exciting professionally but made me, in certain segments of the community, an instant authority on everything from thumbsucking to how to get rid of an annoying mother-in-law. I was called upon to lecture to PTAs, church groups, and every other kind of group you can imagine, including the YWCA, where a charm course was being given; they wanted me to come for an evening "to integrate the personalities of the students." All in all, it was great fun and got my career as a psychiatrist off to a booming start.

The mid-1940s was also a wonderful time to work on the University of California Student Health Service at Cowell Hospital on the Berkeley campus. Under the leadership of Dr. Saxton Pope, an internist who had become a psychiatrist, the mental health service had just been reorganized and revitalized. A dedicated group of enthusiastic, analytically oriented young professional people from psychiatry, psychology, and psychiatric social work formed a training center that soon became known as one of the best facilities in the area for research and treatment of emotional problems in the student-age group. During that era, this ranged from roughly sixteen to the middle thirties. Returnees from the war, older than the usual college student, were beginning to use their G. I. Bill of Rights to return to the university, and many showed up on our service with a variety of war-related problems, along with younger students having the usual problems of adolescent adjustment. For a while we saw just about every kind of disorder, from the most blatant psychosis to the simplest kind of adolescent confusion. One of the latter that I particularly remember was a beautiful twenty-year-old girl in a state of near panic, who presented herself as an emergency during the Easter vacation because nineteen boys had asked her to marry them, and she just had to choose one before the senior prom, where engaged girls paraded with their fiancés.

For a while, before time pressures became too acute, we also had considerable freedom to determine the duration of any treatment offered and gave much collective thought to developing criteria and techniques for using "ego-oriented" short-term therapy in cases that were more often considered to require long-term treatment. Wednesday morning conferences were exciting experiences, with a number of consultants coming in from among the psychiatrists and analysts practicing in the community, to share ideas and comment on specific cases. Everyone loved every minute of it, worked hard, and considered it a privilege to be included.

I spent approximately a third of my working time there and became part of what we all felt to be a kind of family. Most of us were in analysis at the time, and six of us were seeing the same analyst, which must have been rather hard on Professor Erikson. It certainly created somewhat bizarre "sibling" relationships on our staff, but we were all welded together by shared goals and a high degree of cooperation. We may have had our rivalries, but we also had a lot of empathy for each other, and I think the support of that group through the hard years of my analysis was one of the things that kept me going.

So far as I know, there was no bias against women at Cowell, nor were they accepted only because men were not available. If the war created advantages for us, they came to both men and women on the student health service through the kinds of students brought to the university, introducing a great variety of material for our observation and broadening our therapeutic experience. Although I think that era was the height of its glory, the service maintained a high level of quality for many years. After the death of Dr. Pope, personality clashes on the later staff brought about its deterioration into a humdrum service without distinction. However, during the era in which I worked there it was an inspiring place, and to it I owe much of my later concern with the problems of adolescence.

There is no doubt in my mind that until the past ten or fifteen years, the 1940s were also the most advantageous years for women to become candidates for classical psychoanalytic training—those years when most men had not yet returned from overseas. Maybe a few statistics can tell the tale.

From the founding of the San Francisco Psychoanalytic Institute in 1942 to 1953, twelve women were accepted as candidates, one of whom moved away before graduation. During the whole period between 1945 and June 1982, only fifteen women had graduated. Four of them graduated in the late 1950s and 1960s, all of whom had been accepted in that earlier period. (I myself had first been accepted in 1947 but resigned for a while and was reaccepted later.) Although 10 percent of the 142 graduates of the institute between 1945 and 1982 were women—a reasonable percentage in view of the ratio between men and women doctors in general—80 percent of these women graduates had been accepted as candidates in the early years of the institute, during a period in which we can assume that there were fewer male applicants.

In recent years, of course, things have changed. Of the 80 candidates training in 1984, 13, or 16 percent, were women, more female candidates than there have ever been at any one time, and almost twice the total percentage of women who had graduated in the previous period of nearly forty years.

I applied for analytic training in 1946, primarily because I had decided to go into analysis myself and wanted to work with Erik Erikson, who at that time was a training analyst limiting his practice largely to candidates. That seemed then like a good enough reason to apply, although I later felt much better motivated to become an analyst myself. Erikson had agreed to work with me if the committee accepted me, and they did. I still can't figure out why. From what I have since learned about the kind of person thought suitable for training, I was far too anxious and confused in my personal life to be considered a good bet. I feel reasonably sure that if I had applied a year later I never would have made it. Again I was in the right place at exactly the right time.

During those first five years in practice, my interests were still somewhat split between psychiatry and pediatrics. As part of the health department program, I was running a demonstration clinic for nurses in which I was trying to show the important role of both doctor and nurse in recognizing potential emotional problems in children and helping to prevent them by relieving the anxieties of parents. In private practice I was also working with some disturbed children, but I soon found that helping their parents deal with their own anxieties was the biggest part of the job. I particularly remember two such cases that I saw in those earliest days, one in the clinic and the other in my office.

A young Southern girl, who couldn't have been over seventeen, brought her baby to the clinic because he was spitting up all his feedings. It was immediately obvious why this was happening. The mother held him clenched across the stomach, laid across her lap with his head tilted down, and was jabbing the bottle in and out in such a way that every time the baby got a good suck on the nipple it was immediately yanked out again. As soon as the nurse or I held him, he drank perfectly well without regurgitating. However, there was no use in just telling the mother she wasn't holding the baby properly; she was so upset and defensive and scared of being blamed for the baby's problem that all she could hear was criticism. We had to work with her for quite a while to gain her confidence before any suggestions could be made. We simply had to talk to her and find out why she was so anxious.

The girl lived in an overcrowded housing project for shipyard workers, sharing a small two-room apartment with her parents and a girlfriend who had come to visit but stayed on because she had a boyfriend "courtin'." Tensions were running high in everyone. There was nothing I could do about that for the moment, because she insisted the situation couldn't be changed, but what I could and did do was have her come to the clinic twice a week for a while, ostensibly to check the baby's weight but actually to let her ventilate and to encourage whatever efforts she made with the baby. It was not very long before she held him in a much more relaxed way and had somehow managed to get her girlfriend out of the place. Miraculously the baby stopped "spittin' " and began to gain weight. The mother came in regularly thereafter, followed all our advice, and the baby did fine. I saw him last as a three-year-old with no feeding problems or any other evidence of disturbance.

Another young mother came to me privately about her five-year-old son, who had eneuresis. She was very upset about it and wanted me to take the child into treatment, but I said, "Before we make any decisions about that, I'd like to get a little acquainted with you." That was the last word I had a chance to say to her for the next six weeks. She came in once a week, sat down, and talked steadily about herself and her own childhood.

As a child, this woman had always wanted to be a little golden-haired Mary Pickford rather than the dark, scrawny, non-princess that she was, and her first child turned out to be exactly what she had dreamed of being. Just before her son was born, her adored and idealized daughter was killed in an automobile accident. The mother had been devastated. She talked about this for several weeks until she stopped right in the middle and said, "I wonder if I've been trying to make this boy into the daughter I lost?" I said, "Maybe so. Let's talk a little bit about the boy now." She laughed and said, "Oh, he's fine. Hasn't wet the bed for four weeks." I don't know whether that mother solved all her ambivalences about her dead daughter, but she solved that boy's problem for the moment, which is what she came for.

Things aren't always so simple, of course, but I had had a certain amount of experience in working with people's anxieties before I began doing intensive psychotherapy, and it helped shape my ideas on therapeutic techniques.

I think it is fortunate that a good many of my attitudes toward doing psychotherapy were formed before I entered analytic training. Perhaps it is heresy to be glad about that, but I am, nevertheless. Most of my training was psychoanalytically oriented, but my first teacher was Stanislaus Szurek on the Langley Porter Children's Service, who, although an analyst himself, had a horror of using analytic lingo. I picked up from him the idea that if you can't explain in English what you are doing, you don't understand it, and the use of technical terms in therapy just confuses people. Szurek called himself a nondirective therapist. (He really wasn't, although he may not have recognized how much directing he did with his eyebrows.) In any case, he taught nondirectiveness, and he taught me a great many things that are still pretty much the basis of the way I think about therapy even thirty-five years later.

One of the first things he taught me was that it wasn't my job to tell people anything; my job was to hear what the patients told me. He taught me to listen for what the patient wants and try to understand what is interfering with his or her ability to attain a particular goal. Without ever using the words *transference* or *counter-transference*, he also taught me that the best way to understand the patient was to observe the interaction between us and use my understanding of that interaction to help the patient understand his or her ways of dealing with others. That was back in 1946. Nowadays a lot of analysts are treating that concept of working with the interaction as though it were something new, but that's the way I was taught by Szurek way back then. I haven't always done it, but I have often been sorry that I didn't.

Szurek also drummed into me something that surely has been told to everyone trained in clinical work—the notion that the therapist should not impose his or her idea of what is good for the patient on the patient, nor should he or she be thinking about somebody else when dealing with a patient. This sounds elementary—"Keep your eye on the ball and remember who is your patient." But it isn't always easy, and a lot of people who ought to know better pay no attention to it. This may be particularly difficult when working on a children's service.

People who work on a children's service tend to be child-oriented, and if a therapist sees something going on between a mother and a child, the therapist is apt to consider the welfare of the child first, even if the mother is the patient. If the therapist is constantly thinking about the good of the child, it will interfere with the mother's therapy. I had this beaten into me early, and I'm very glad I did because it has come up a number of times in my practice when there was a great temptation to forget it.

One young woman came into my office with the chief complaint that she had impulses to kill her infant daughter. Her life was extremely chaotic. Her husband had told her that he was homosexual and had gone off to live with a man. She herself had subsequently gotten into a mutually clinging sort of relationship with a lesbian woman, and at the time she came to me, she looked as though she was going to fall apart. My first impression was that this was a horrible situation in which to bring up a child and that perhaps my treatment goal should be to help her give up the child for adoption. But then that little voice in the back of my head started talking: "This woman has come to you for help with her own impulses. She is your patient. After all, she is concerned enough about the child to come for treatment." And so I started to work with her around the problem for which she wanted help.

I found out that she herself had been brought up by a psychotic mother who beat her. I can't remember all the details now, but it became obvious that all this was what she was afraid of repeating with the child, for whom she actually had a lot of warm feelings. We worked together for a long time, she straightened out her life, and she now has a pretty good relationship with her daughter. If I had decided to act upon what I thought would be best for the child I would not have been a very good therapist for the mother, and I am quite sure the outcome for the child would have been very much worse.

Another woman came to me who was a twin. She had had an unsuccessful marriage to a man who didn't want children, but she was nearing forty and was extremely anxious to have a child while there was still time. Her twin sister had been married for a long time and had several children, and the patient decided that she wanted to get pregnant even if she couldn't find another man she wanted to marry. Her mother, who was a member of one of the psychological professions, was horrified, and was paying for the treatment in the hope that it would dissuade her daughter from this plan.

After talking to this woman for a short time, it seemed evident to me that her desperate desire to have a child was due to a feeling of being incomplete without her twin sister and that having a child with this kind of motivation would not be good for either mother or child.

However, again I had to ask myself, "Is it my job to protect this baby from being born, or is it my job to help this woman clarify her own thinking about what she wants?" I also had to remember that it was not my job to satisfy the patient's mother, who was paying for the treatment, but to help my patient understand her own motivations and then make up her own mind without pressure from me one way or the other. We went ahead on this basis, and when it was all over, she went ahead and had the child. I was left with the feeling that I hadn't done a very good piece of therapy, but now, many years later, she has done a splendid job as a mother and has a lovely daughter. Would she have been better off if I had managed to impose my own view on her, and deprived her of a chance for motherhood? In the future She may have difficulties along the way, as most people do, but one can at least hope that she learned she can get help when she feels she needs it.

For the first few years my interest was about equally divided between working directly with children in play therapy and working with parents whose children were having problems. However, I began to realize that although some of the children I saw had symptoms arising from internalized earlier experiences and were living in relatively stable current home situations, many of them had symptoms related to disturbances in current relationships with their parents. I found that those symptoms often cleared up dramatically when their parents were helped. I gradually became more interested in adults seeking help for their own problems, and in that early period, tended to choose as patients, parents, teachers and others in a position to influence children. This often in volved more long-term, intensive exploration of mental conflict, and as I saw more people who were deeply disturbed in various ways, I became more fascinated with learning to understand the ways in which their minds worked. Perhaps this interest was fostered by the fact that I could see the progress of schizophrenia in my own brother, and probably may being in analysis myself helped it along. but beyond that, I think I had always had a great curiosity to know the whys of things. I wanted more training in understanding and dealing with psychotic people, and incidentally needed three more months of training to satisfy the requirements for Psychiatric Boards. The question was how to get it, and when.

          ✳ The year 1950 was a turbulent time in Berkeley, not only for me but for a great many other people as well. Struggles over the loyalty oath had disrupted the university and created great conflict for everyone involved. Our staff at Cowell Hospital had offered to resign in a body but were told that there were already enough prominent non-signers, and nobody wanted martyrs. This left us to make individual choices over whether we felt strongly enough to quit our jobs without support. Most of us didn't, although we were against the oath and felt wracked by conflict and guilt. As in any civil war, friends were alienated over the issue and misery reigned. Erikson, in sympathy with the non-signers, had already achieved fame by writing *Childhood* and *Society*—and was leaving for the East to divide his time between Austen-Riggs Foundation in Massachusetts and a professorship at the University of Pittsburgh. I had reached a point in my analysis where it was feasible to interrupt and wasn't ready to think about going on with anyone else. Above all, I was in the throes of trying to make a decision about whether or not to get married.

    I had finally met a man whom I had grown to love very much—a man totally unlike anyone with whom I had ever been involved before. I think my analysis had made this possible. Leland Vaughan was a charming, quiet man with a keen sense of humor and an ability to enjoy life—a man who was loyal, totally reliable, and absolutely honest. I admired him deeply as well as loved him. What I felt was not the stormy fascination I had felt for Rory but a warm, steady love and sense of total security in being loved. In everything I consider important we saw eye to eye, but in many ways we were quite different, and I feared the impact of those differences on both of us.

    He was both an artist and a practical man who liked to work with his hands—a gifted designer, at home in the outdoors and a respected professor of landscape architecture at the University of California—but not a would-be intellectual and lover of talk, like myself. Would he continue to care for a woman "whose idea of camping is to turn your electric blanket down to medium?" I loved the outdoors too, but I also liked my comforts and became impatient away from civilization for any length of time. I needed the stimulation of play with ideas, an occupation that tended to make him uncomfortable. Although I wanted to be more like him, I was a more restless person and felt I might not be easy for him to live with. I felt that what he loved about me were aspects of my mother—qualities that he saw as feminine and a certain vulnerability requiring the support of his masculine strength. Would he continue to love a successful doctor, and a psychiatrist to boot? I wasn't sure, and I didn't think he was either. It seemed like a good time to take a break and give ourselves time to see how we felt after a period of separation.

At that period, the Commonwealth Fund was offering fellowships for pediatricians to get training in psychiatry, and I was eligible in view of my ongoing well-baby work at the health department. Still dangling between my two lines of interest, I applied for a year's support to spend half time each at the Yale Psychiatric Institute and the Child Study Center in New Haven under Dr. Milton Senn, with whom I was now pretty well acquainted. They gave it to me, and although things didn't work out quite as I had planned, a whole new vista opened up before me. The year in New Haven turned out to be two, and some of it wasn't easy, but the things I did there and the friends I made helped turn the whole direction of my career from its former course.

Three months before I left, and on the very day I had told all my patients I would be leaving, my brother chose to enter his New World too, and committed suicide.

New Haven and Back

There just never was time to mourn my brother. In the next three months I not only had to take care of all his affairs but had to see about renting my house, make arrangements for the referral of all my patients, and listen to their complaints about feeling abandoned. I knew what that was like, having just been through it myself at the announcement of Erikson's imminent departure, but I had to go over it all again with them, each and every one of them. There were only three months in which to do all that and to arrange leaves of absence from my jobs and make arrangements for others to take over. Only three months to tie up the loose ends in my own life, find homes for my cats, say goodbye to my friends, and reconcile myself to a year away from the man I now loved but wasn't sure I wanted to marry.

One thing that kept me going was the prospect of both regression and progression. In a sense I would be going home for a while, to territory within an hour's drive from Bloomfield. For a time I could sink my roots again in New England soil and find a kind of peace. At the same time, I was going forward professionally as an experienced member of the psychiatric community, with a desirable fellowship as testimony to a respectable reputation. To myself and everyone else, I would be a person with a purpose. In the past, change of scene had always been a gesture of uncertainty and insecurity. This change was voluntary and temporary, with a firm knowledge of what I was moving toward and assurance of a home base to which I could return. I was sad about leaving but also felt a certain excited anticipation. That was until I arrived in New Haven.

Advanced trainees in the department of psychiatry at Yale were usually placed on state hospital service, coming to YPI (the Yale Psychiatric Institute) only for seminars and conferences. That is the way I had expected to spend three to six months, with the rest of my stay spent on the children's service at the Child Study Center under Dr. Senn. When I got there, however, I found that the YPI hospital itself was short of staff, and the department had decided to use me there full-time along with four first-year residents. This was contrary to the contract and was not what the Commonwealth Fund had agreed to, but that's the way it would have been had I not protested vigorously against being exploited. I was forced into a knock-down, drag-out fight with the head of the department, who didn't care much for female psychiatrists anyway, and certainly didn't like to be challenged by one. We finally compromised with an agreement by which I stayed at YPI with only a half load of patients and permission to take part in a number of research projects at CSC. Actually this was a satisfactory arrangement for my purposes, but the whole altercation left a bad taste in my mouth from the start and soured my feeling about the department in particular and the whole venture in general.

There I was—suddenly, in effect, reduced to the position of a first-year trainee, years older than my co-workers, with all my peer group in the ranks of professors, stripped of status in a strange environment, angry, lonely, and increasingly anxious. I tried to be a good sport about it because I really was getting most of what I had come for, but the anger and frustration apparently touched off a whole load of feelings that had just been biding their time to explode.

An emotional reaction to my brother's death had hitherto remained precariously suppressed, but now it hit me with full force. Throughout my first six months in New Haven tension mounted. All the grief and anxiety over his suicide overflowed, and all the ancient guilts and ambivalences toward him, which had been partially resolved in analysis, were now revived with full emotional impact, precipitated by the fear that my decision to leave California had made final his own wish to leave this world. Was his act carried out as a reproach to me? A previous aborted attempt had been made a year earlier on my birthday, and this one on the day I finally committed myself absolutely to going away. Had my relative success been too much for his fragile self-esteem? Was our closeness in recent years merely a cover-up for deep-seated jeaiousy and hatred? Was I to blame for his problems simply by having been born in the first place? All these questions whirled around in my head accompanied by crushing sorrow—sorrow for him, for me, and for our whole unhappy family. I went about my work barely holding back tears most of the time.

I believe that my own emotional stability was at least partly restored by working with an adolescent girl named Patty. Patty was a catatonic schizophrenic who had been in the hospital for over a year without speaking a word or allowing any doctor to make contact with her. Talking to her had proved useless, as I found out myself when I tried, but perhaps because I had worked with children, I thought that something in the nature of play therapy might be a possible approach. I bought her a doll and started making a few tentative comments to it. This worked like a charm. Patty still didn't speak, but the doll responded to my remarks by nodding or shaking its head, and pretty soon Patty and I had estabhished a fairly good system of communication. As we went along, her whole expression brightened, she looked healthier, and there were quite a few changes in her behavior on the ward. After a while she even occasionally uttered a word or two in the exclusive presence of the ward aide who was responsible for most of her care, and who was very fond of her. It really looked as though things were moving, and I was delighted. I presented an account of our work together as a continuous case to Dr. William Pious, a local authority on the treatment of schizophrenia, and he was delighted. He suggested that I present it to the whole group of students and staff, who also seemed to be delighted.

In the course of all this, a good portion of my self-esteem was restored, I regained my lost status as an experienced therapist, and I laid the foundation for a thirty-year friendship with Drs. Theodore and Ruth Lidz, who had devoted most of their careers to work with schizophrenic patients. The experience solidified my interest in doing psychotherapy with this kind of patient and led to my becoming involved in a research study on families of schizophrenic patients which Dr. Theodore Lidz and the co-workers who stayed with it published as a book some time afterward (*Schizophrenia and the Family, 1965*). In fact, it was the first step toward a whole new set of interests.

For Patty the outcome was not so fortunate. Just at a point where everyone felt hopeful that she might eventually get better, her family ran out of funds to keep her in a private hospital, and one afternoon, without warning to either me or Patty, she was whisked away to a state hospital, where she probably got a prefrontal lobotomy. That was the treatment for "hopeless" patients in those days, before antipsychotic drugs could sometimes restore people to a semblance of functioning, and that's what probably happened to her unless she was simply tucked away on a back ward and forgotten.

Thirty years later, I still feel angry about the brutal way that whole affair was handled—snapping without warning the first fragile threads of trust Patty had ever spun. But the truth is that even if she had remained at YPI, I was not prepared to forfeit my own life to stay and continue her treatment as long as might have been necessary, and I have to face the fact that within a year she would have had to deal with an abandonment that could have been just as devastating if not more so. Fate is not kind to people in Patty's condition, and even today, unless their families can afford to keep them in one of the country's very few good long-term treatment centers, the outlook for their future is not good, drugs or no drugs.

One other patient contributed significantly to my professional growth by setting me to thinking about a kind of interaction between parents and children that had received little attention in the psychiatric world—one that I later found to be common in a certain segment of society and wrote about in a number of articles. The interaction was one for which I coined the name "masked authoritarianism." The patient was a boy named Jake whom I saw as a private patient for three months during the summer.

Jake was a freshman at a prestigious college, who had had to drop out after suddenly developing an acute learning block. As he hoped to return in the fall, we had a maximum of three months available to cure the symptom if possible, but he was willing to come for treatment every day during that period. Both he and his father, who brought him, were highly motivated to cooperate, and I decided to experiment with a greatly condensed form of intensive treatment. Jake and I met alone for quite a while, then I met with the father alone and finally with both of them together in a couple of highly emotional sessions. The boy's symptoms disappeared, and although I advised him to continue therapy at a later time, he had gotten what he came for.

Jake had grown up during the era in which "permissive" child-rearing was much in vogue, particularly among well-educated, liberal families. His father, a progressive, intellectual professional man, had himself been raised by a very authoritarian old-world father and had been determined not to make the mistakes with his son that he felt his father had made with him. He wanted the boy to think for himself and make his own decisions from an early age. Unfortunately, he often did not feel as permissive as he wanted to act, and although he was quite unaware of what he was doing, he carried on a kind of rule by indirection. He brought his son up to believe that to be a man meant to be able to make his own decisions, but every time the boy made a decision the father didn't like, he let his disappointment in Jake's judgment show. On the other hand, whenever the boy chose something he approved, he gave him great praise for the ability to make a correct choice—that is, to be a real man. Jake loved his father and thought of him as truly permissive, but unconsciously he perceived the manipulation and felt his sense of manhood threatened. All anger toward such a "good" father had to be repressed from awareness but found expression through the development of symptoms.

When Jake and his father became aware of how they had been in-teracting, both of them expressed intense emotion, after which the boy got over his block. Later, back in Berkeley, the home of liberal intel-lectuals from authoritarian backgrounds, I found this kind of interaction rife not only between parents and children but also between teachers and pupils at all levels of the academic system. I have come to feel that it sometimes occurs also between analyst and patient. It has never been widely recognized, but awareness of it has been extremely useful to me in many aspects of my work. Jake and his father taught me about it, and to them, as to Gordon and Patty, I feel I owe an important aspect of my own education.

During the summer after that first year in New Haven, Leland came out for a long visit during which we got a lot of things ironed out and definitely decided to get married. He managed to convince me that although he did indeed value my "femininity," he wasn't looking for a dependent, fluffy little wife and was quite capable of handling his feelings about being the husband of a psychiatrist. I convinced him that I didn't need him to become more verbal and valued him just the way he was. Heaven forbid that I should be married to a masculine counterpart of myself! Before we finished talking, both of us were sure we understood each other and could discuss any problems we might encounter.

Before that visit I hadn't been quite sure and had made a commitment to spend another year of half-time research on the family project with Dr. Lidz. After the visit, I became restless to get back to California and begin a new phase of my life. Both Leland and I found it hard to prolong our separation, but the time passed eventually, and I never regretted spending the extra year at Yale.

In those two years I had good opportunities to learn more about children in two research seminars with the famous psychoanalyst Ernst Kris and later, under the direction of Dr. Senn, as part-time consultant to an old-fashioned orphanage that was trying to modernize into a children's treatment center. It was all excellent experience, but before the end of my stay, I had already made the decision to finish my analytic training and work full-time with disturbed adults.

✻ Upon return to Berkeley, I gave up my identification with pediatrics and child psychiatry. The insights I had gained from working with children in various capacities had been and continued to be of great value in every other aspect of my professional growth, but from that time on, my primary interest lay in other areas. Although for a number of years I continued my consultation and teaching in the field of public health, most of the last thirty-five years of my professional life have been devoted to private practice, in which my time has been about evenly divided between treating schizophrenic or borderline adolescents and treating more neurotic adults through psychoanalysis or modifications of it.

I should like to think it is generally true that learning continues throughout the whole of one's professional career. I know that it did for me. During those years of practice, two analysts had a major influence on my work—two of the best conceptual thinkers I have ever encountered. One was Dr. Mary Sarvis, with whom I shared an office and enjoyed an ongoing exchange of ideas over coffee twice a day for nearly twenty years. Unfortunately she died before achieving the national recognition that she deserved, but we offered each other a kind of stimulation that was invaluable to me. The other was Dr. Merton Gill whom I first knew at Yale and later during his years in Berkeley. He, fortunately, did achieve his deserved status as a leading theorist and teacher in the field of psychoanalysis. My respect for his integrity and courage as teacher, analyst, consultant and friend knows no bounds, and I consider it a privilege to have had close contact over the years with his way of thinking which has had a significant effect on my own.

6 Marriage

From the age of five, when his mother reprimanded his older brother for calling him "that little punk," Punk became the ineradicable nickname by which Leland Vaughan was known throughout the rest of his life. Everyone called him that, from the president of the University of California down to his smallest grandchild. Most people didn't even know what his given name was, but as soon as they got over the immediate shock, everyone who knew him completely forgot whatever other connotations "punk" had for them and used the nickname as a term of endearment. To almost everyone with whom he came in contact, male or female, Punk was a very endearing man.

We were married six months after my return from New Haven and laughed about our wedding all the way down to a Palm Springs honeymoon. As neither of us was affiliated with any church, we had arranged to be married quietly at home by a Unitarian minister who agreed to perform the ceremony without having met us beforehand. He arrived promptly, sitting down with us and the witnesses for what we thought was to be a short chat to get acquainted. As the time stretched on and on, however, it suddenly began to dawn on us that he thought we were the parents of a bride and groom who were to arrive. When informed that the bride and groom had indeed arrived, the poor young man was so flustered he could barely stagger through the ceremony. We nearly disrupted it ourselves with attempts to avoid a fit of giggles. Punk and

I tended to become hilarious over events that others saw as only mildly funny.

We did a good deal of laughing together in the course of our marriage but also shared a lot of sorrows, particularly in our earliest years together. During the first five years, while not yet entirely recovered from the death of my brother, I lost both parents, my sister, and my close friend Jay, with whom I had shared an apartment in the old New York days. Punk helped me weather those losses, but when my turn came to help him, I don't think I did quite as well. The death of his oldest son, in an automobile accident which completely devastated Punk, opened so many old wounds in me that I fell apart as well, and I don't think either of us ever totally recovered.

During those early years, both of us had to do make great efforts to adjust to everything that required adjustment. Three months after our marriage, Punk's former wife died, and his boys, Steve, fifteen, and Nick, twelve, came to live with us full-time. Two young boys who had just lost their mother returned to live in the house where they had spent their early childhood, and now had to adjust to sharing their father with a relative stranger. Practically overnight I had not only to become a wife for the first time at the age of forty, but to assume probably the most difficult role with which any woman can hope to cope—that of a stepmother to teenagers. I had to make a rapid shift from the role of therapist to that of parent, which isn't easy to do. The boys father had to assume the hardest role of all, that of trying to pay attention to all our needs and keep everyone reasonably happy while still carrying on an exacting job at the university. This situation required a great deal of effort on all our parts, and we all tried hard.

The image I have now, as I think back to those first few weeks, is of shoes—huge shoes dropped off in a trail across the living room from the front door. I guess that image needs no explanation, but it wasn't only shoes. It was huge down jackets and school books and balls and fishing gear, including half-opened bait jars full of rotten abalone guts, all over what had been a relatively neat and orderly house. I felt almost overwhelmed by the raw maleness with which I was suddenly surrounded, after a life led almost entirely in the company of women. In some ways I was delighted to be at last part of a family sharing the casual indoor-outdoor life style in which a good many California children are reared, but I wasn't used to it. In fact, I had been somewhat compulsive about neatness, and although I was determined not to inflict this on the others, the clutter bothered me. I don't think I showed it, as with apparent aplomb I simply collected the shoes and jackets and piled them in the hall, but it took a certain toll in emotional energy.

In spite of this, I didn't anticipate any real trouble in learning to handle the situation. After all, I had been fairly successful in my relationships with adolescents, hadn't I? I had chosen to work professionally with adolescent boys because I liked them, and most of them had liked me. I was highly trained in recognizing their needs and feelings and was pretty well up on current fads and lingo. Why shouldn't I be able to do as well with my own stepchildren as I had done with my patients?

Of one thing I was sure: I wasn't going to make the same kinds of mistakes I had seen made by others in the same position. No, sir! Not me! I knew all the pitfalls, and I wasn't going to step into any of them. First and foremost, I wasn't going to act like a therapist in my own family. I had talked with too many children of mental health professionals who expressed fears that "Daddy" or "Mommy" could read their minds, or felt that pressure to reveal feelings all the time was an invasion of their privacy. I would avoid that at all costs. What's more, I would certainly avoid setting up any conflict of loyalties between me and their own mother. Vivid in my mind was the memory of the wife in an interracial couple who could not tolerate the refusal of her husband's sons to call her "Mother." Vivid also was the image of a young step-mother from an elite segment of Eastern society who, with the best intentions in the world, tried to instill her social and cultural values into children reared in a small central California valley town. I wasn't going to do that either. If the boys' table manners needed correction or their clothes seemed inappropriate for a particular occasion, I would leave it to their father to straighten the situation out. Knowing that they would need time to accept me as having a role in their lives, I would neither reprimand them nor "seduce" them with expressions of physical affection they might not be able to handle. I was analyzed, wasn't I? I certainly knew all the dangers of doing that. All in all, my goal was to be "understanding," friendly, and non-intrusive, demonstrating by every word and deed that I wanted only to be their good friend and had no intention of coming between them and their father. I would wait for them to come to me with whatever affection they could eventually develop. Great resolutions? And I tried very hard to act accordingly.

For his part, my husband was perfectly willing to assume responsibility for all discipline and whatever bodily care or advice might be necessary. He planned expeditions and camping trips that the "men" could enjoy together and did what little chauffeuring was required for boys of that age. We hired a part-time helper to clean house and have dinner ready for us, converged in the evening, and during the day went about our respective jobs and schoolwork with little friction. Under these circumstances, the boys were well behaved and compliant, continued to do well in school, and carried on their usual activities with friends. It looked as though all of us had it made.

By this time I had had years of experience as a psychiatrist. I was probably as good at my job as any of my colleagues, yet it never crossed my mind to ask myself whether, under the circumstances, things might be going a little too well. How many parents, even professionals in the field, spontaneously worry about the fact that their teenagers are giving them no trouble? I think if any other parent had described the situation to me I would at least have raised that question, but with my own family it never entered my head. I had read a lot of books and talked to a lot of people; I had thought a lot and planned a lot and had presumably covered all the angles from the start. But it simply did not occur to me that the boys, who had always been good boys, were being a little too good in this very trying situation. What I did think was that I had learned what it takes to be a good stepmother, that I had tried my best to put that knowledge into action, and that I had accomplished what I set out to do.

As a matter of fact, to some extent I think I did, because in the end things worked out pretty well. I eventually did gain the confidence of both boys and am still a good friend to the one who survived and became a fine man. However, in retrospect I can see that the development of those relationships took far longer than it should have, and the reason it did was in great part my fault. I don't say it was all my fault, because it wasn't, but it was largely due to the fact that all my attempts to be "understanding" grossly interfered with my ability to be spontaneous in relating to those boys—that and an old hang-up of my own.

Maybe you can scrub a pot clean if you work at it enough, but when you try to scrape a psyche clean with psychoanalysis, it seems that stubborn bits almost inevitably cling to the sides. In this case, what hung me up was my old childhood problem, now masquerading under the guise of an intellectual decision not to intrude into a close family group. It was my almost fatalistic tendency to accept being neither in nor out.

I can see now that I never let anyone know how much I wanted to be in on that tight little family threesome, and I think I was far too cautious and withdrawn from participation in their closeness. My wish to avoid intruding came across to them as lack of involvement and caused everyone to preserve a distance that could have been reduced much sooner than it was. Everyone paid a certain price for family tensions that could have been avoided, or at least been less prolonged. Anyway, that's what I think now.

In retrospect it is obvious that the boys were indeed too good, because they felt they had to be. They were not sure enough of what my reaction would be if they made any waves. What young people can really feel safe with a parental figure who never criticizes or gets mad; who never gives them an opportunity to get mad or blow up and then be forgiven with a hug and a pat on the back? How can they know that their father's new wife really feels affectionate toward them if all she expresses is a friendly neutrality? How can they know that all her knowledge of the pitfalls has caused her to step into the biggest pitfall of all?

Of course, there is no way to know whether things would have gone better if I hadn't had these problems. I have seen ghastly outcomes to situations where a stepmother has gone with her feelings and tried to move too quickly into the bosom of an unready family or has tried to force physical affection on hostile children. A stepmother always walks a narrow path between being overintrusive and abdicating too much of her rightful role as mother-substitute, and has to play it by ear, learning as she goes along.

I finally learned a lot of things, and learned them the hard way. How I wish now that I could have felt free enough to risk "seducing" them with an occasional hug, even if in so doing I also risked being pushed away! I am pretty sure it wouldn't have hurt any, and it might have helped a lot.

After a few years, Steve went off to college in the East and Nick to boarding school near his brother. Punk and I were finally alone together. I was at the height of my career and he at the height of his, looking forward to an early retirement after all the stress of being temporary dean of his college during the stressful years of student unrest and political uprisings. He was on the board of the International Federation of Landscape Architects, which met almost every year in a different foreign country, so for a while we traveled abroad a lot or drove all around the western United States, picknicking and camping as we went along. Later, when Nick married young and became a father himself, we became involved with grandchildren who lived right next door for a while. Unfortunately, shortly after his much anticipated retirement, Punk became ill and died two years later

In restrospect, I see the years of our marriage as a wonderful time in my life—years that made everything else worthwhile. They were twenty full, active years—years full of ups and downs but on the whole happy ones for me, and I think for him, in spite of the shadow cast upon him by losing Steve.

Although we were quite different in many ways, we had been completely together on all the things I consider important. We both loved our home on the Bay with its beautiful garden that he had designed. We loved our cabin on the Sonoma Coast, which he had built with his own hands. He taught me to appreciate problems facing the environment—to know the plants, wild birds, whales migrating, and seals playing on the rocks. To him the stuff of life was being close to nature, and often we sat together for long stretches of time without saying a word, just listening to the wind in the pines over our heads and waves dashing against the rocky cliffs below. Sometimes I would become restless in the silences and once complained that he didn't talk more about his thoughts and feelings. He looked at me in astonishment and said, "But you know how I feel, and I know how you feel! Why should we have to talk about it?" He was right, of course. He wasn't as verbal as I am or given to discussing things just for the sake of the discussion, but when he did say something, he had thought carefully about the subject and presented lies views with infinite reasonableness.

Leland Vaughan was steady as a rock and totally reliable. He didn't know much about psychological theories and didn't want to, but he knew people and often gave me useful, commonsense comments on the problems I occasionally brought home from the office. His values were the same as mine on philosophy of life, sexuality, and sense of humor. The activities we enjoyed and the people we enjoyed being with were often quite different, but we had a shared group of friends with whom we both felt comfortable. We loved to travel together, but driving along the roads or sitting in sidewalk cafés, we each saw different aspects of the scenery or the social scene. Fortunately for us both, we respected our differences and did not try to change each other's views. For over twenty years, leading lives that were sometimes separate, sometimes shared, we were close emotionally until the day he died.

I was past sixty at that time and felt that my life was essentially over in spite of the long-living genes within me. I planned to continue my professional work, enjoy my grandchildren, and serve out my time as best I could with those of my friends who still remained. The part of my life that mattered to me was gone, and I did not expect to replace it. However, Fate had other plans for me, and after six years of widowhood, I married again and started a whole new kind of relationship.

My present husband is Otto Will, a man of stature in my own profession with whom I had had some professional contact from time to time. He is brilliant, verbal, and eclectic in his interests, filling our house with books on many aspects of natural science, cosmology, and philosophy as well as psychology, poetry, and fiction. He loves to discuss things and also has a playful side that I find delightful. He furnishes a constant influx of surprises—flowers and cartoon books, wind-up mechanical toys and Southwest Indian fetishes. I never know quite what is going to happen next.

In his younger days, Otto was also a man of the outdoors, climbing the beloved mountain peaks of his native Colorado, driving his tractor in Maryland, or cross-country skiing in the Berkshires, where he spent eleven years as medical director of the Austen-Riggs Foundation. He swears it isn't so, but I am sure that some of his happiest days were spent in active service with the Navy on an outmoded, ill-equipped ship in the South Pacific during the war. You can't hear him tell stories about that period without feeling his excitement and knowing he loved every minute of it.

Otto is now seventy-six but still wields a chain saw on recalcitrant shrubbery and chops kindling wood with gusto. He still loves the outdoors, but his way of life is not and never has been similar to that of my first husband. I wouldn't want it to be. He is an entirely different person—impulsive, moody, and often quite unpredictable along with all his other wonderful qualities, and the way we relate to each other is not the same although we love each other, are good for each other, and have many mutual interests and activities. He too is uncompetitive with me and actually seems to take more pride in my accomplishments than he does in his own, which are far greater.

I don't know how things would have gone if we had married thirty years ago. I suspect that I would have been tempted to shine by reflected light and that the suppression of my own competitiveness would have been damaging to us both. He would never have had the children who now mean so much to him, and I think it likely that we would have been far less emotionally close than we now are in our seventies. As it is, we live a quiet life in great harmony, and I have a whole new set of stepchildren—fortunately this time grownup stepchildren—to enjoy.

7 Forty Years in Private Practice

On Professional Writing

On a warm, sunny Sunday in the spring of 1955, a colleague from Cowell Hospital invited me for an afternoon at his swimming pool to meet a distinguished visitor from the East. What a wonderful invitation that was! The visitor was Dr. Frieda Fromm-Reichmann, a famous psychoanalyst whose books I had studied and used as a basis for much of my own thinking about treating severely disturbed patients. She was one of the people I most admired in the field, and now she was coming up from the Center for Advanced Studies at Palo Alto, where she was spending a year in research, for a leisurely "family" afternoon in the Wheelrights' garden. To me it was like being asked to spend an informal afternoon with Eleanor Roosevelt at the White House. I arrived in a state of reverence and awe, which, however, did not last long. The famous doctor and our hostess were already bobbing around in the pool and waved for me to join them as though I were an old chum. Thus a new chapter in my life began.

Nearly thirty years later it is hard to remember exactly what happened next. What I do remember, and will remember all my life, is that within a very short time all three of us were deep in conversation about the ways in which unconscious ideas manifest themselves symbolically. You would have to have been there to believe it—three little middle-aged ladies floating lazily around the blue water of a shining pool, surrounded by flowering spring and talking about primary process! It could only happen in Marin County, California. For quite a while we floated and bobbed around and talked a blue streak, having the time of our lives. Before we emerged from that pool, it seemed as though I had known Frieda Fromm-Reichmann forever.

Throughout that afternoon and well into the evening, we talked on about what interested everyone in the group, which included two Jungian analysts, an authority on the psychotherapy of schizophrenia, and I, who had recently worked with the Lidzes in New Haven on a study of families of schizophrenic patients. It was one of the most stimulating days I can remember, and in the course of it, I told them about some unusual material I was collecting in therapy with a disturbed six-teen-year-old boy who used a symbolic language to talk about universal adolescent problems. Everyone seemed interested, but Dr. Fromm-Reichmann particularly so. Before we broke up, she asked me to send her a copy of the notes and to plan to go over them with her on my next trip to Washington. She really meant it! She wasn't just being polite! It took me a while to convince myself of that, but funally, in an anguish of ambivalence, and feeling rather foolish, I did it. Not long afterward, I turned up at Chestnut Lodge, where she lived and worked, and after almost a whole day together discussing my material, she encouraged me to write a book.

In that little cottage, on the grounds of a famous mental hospital, *My Language Is Me* was conceived, a first of its kind. Frieda Fromm-Reichmann was to have been its godmother, but unfortunately she didn't live to see it born. I never realized how truly generous she had been until years later, when I learned that she herself had hoped to write a somewhat similar book in collaboration with a patient of her own, who also used symbolic language. That book, later written as fiction by the patient herself, became the famous *I Never Promised You a Rose Garden*.

Long before I ever met Dr. Fromm-Reichmann, in fact back in my medical school days, one thing had already become very obvious to me. This was that even the most learned and inspired teachers often failed to impress their students as much as an article that somebody had considered worthy of publication in a scientific journal. "Get it into the literature if you want to be heard!" I had long since become convinced of that and had already published a number of short articles in psychoanalytic journals and a monograph for the U.S. Department of Health and Welfare about the Berkeley health department program. However, the idea of writing a book had never occurred to me except as a kind of fantasy; that I could write a scientific book seemed like a megalomanic delusion.

The way I saw it, good professional books offer new theories, and although I felt that the most distinguished members of my profession concerned themselves with speculations at that level, I never considered myself either capable of or interested in doing so. I considered myself pretty good at analyzing material and drawing conclusions from my own observations, but theorizing at higher levels of abstraction wasn't my thing. If I ever made a contribution to the field, it would be as a teacher who had a certain knack for making abstract ideas intelligible to those who, like myself, can grasp them better when translated into simple English, illustrated by clear, concrete examples.

One of the things that fascinated me most in clinical practice was relating what I heard from patients to the theories I had read—getting the evidence to substantiate the abstract ideas. Psychotherapy and analysis give one the opportunity to hear what actually goes on between people—to learn the details of life and behavior on which theoretical conclusions are based. That is what appeals to me. I am the Eliza Doolittle of psychiatry—"Words, words, words! Don't tell me about it! *Show* me!" As I have described, the importance of getting the evidence has always impressed me, not only because it was pounded into my head repeatedly by my most highly esteemed teachers, but because there is built into my whole character and approach to life a stubborn need to counteract the kinds of unsubstantiated fantasies masquerading as facts that ran rampant in my family and threatened to addle all our minds.

Then sudden by I was told that one didn't have to be a real theorizer in order to make a genuine contribution to the field—that a play-by-play description of what was actually said and done throughout the whole of a therapeutic relationship between patient and therapist—just the kind of material I had amassed in considerable detail for my own interest—would be valuable for others to see. I didn't have to be a great scientist, and I didn't have to write the Great American Novel. I could describe in a somewhat fictionalized style the interactions in which I had participated and produce something useful to members of my profession. I could be a clinical writer, and it was O.K! For me this opened up a whole world of possibilities.

My therapeutic relationship with the boy was finally concluded, and with his permission, I offered an adaptation of our talks together for publication. The day in 1962 when it was accepted was one of the happiest of my life. I think I felt about that book as I would have felt about having a child. I know it is a cliché to make that equation, but that's the way I felt. That boy and I had together created something that was essentially unique, just as every child is the unique product of its particular parents. Our work together would not only benefit both of us, as it did in different ways, but continue to have a life of its own quite apart from ours, and it would sink or swim by its own merits. There was an exhilaration about that idea which is hard to explain. I have never felt it about anything I achieved subsequently, although I later wrote two more books, one of which got somewhat more public recognition than the first. Just as Frieda Fromm-Reichmann had pushed me into writing *My Language Is Me,* Ted Lidz practically bludgeoned me into writing *A Mingled Yarn.*

While still at Yale in 1952, working on the research about families of schizophrenic patients, I had mentioned to him that I thought descriptions of the interactions between family members failed to give the real flavor of life in such families. I thought someone ought to demonstrate that more graphically and also show how the peculiarities of communication and interaction build up as they pass from one generation to another. I used to tell him stories about my own family—a family with genealogical records and memoirs by members of several generations which illustrated dramatically some of the theoretical points being made in the study. Several of these examples found their way into the book that he and his co-workers later published, but all along, he was pushing me to write that family up myself in such a way as to convey the flavor I was talking about.

At the time I didn't see myself as a writer of anything but prosaic reports and factual journal articles. However, he kept after me through the years, and after publication of *My Language Is Me*, the pressure got so strong that I finally had to do it to get him off my back. That book, a true story written in a somewhat fictionalized style, became *A Mingled Yarn*. In it I tried to paint a picture of what life was like in the family of someone who later became schizophrenic and to give my interpretation of what I had described. Again, it was a more or less play-by-play account of what real people actually said and did. It could be published only because all but one member of the family was dead, and I was willing to allow public scrutiny of my family's peculiarities in the interests of research.

Detailed descriptions and verbatim accounts of what goes on in private between people in a family or in a psychotherapy interview are published rather rarely, for a number of good reasons. In the first place, it takes a certain amount of exhibitionism, or counterphobia, to expose oneself to the close scrutiny of others. A psychotherapist works alone in an office with a single patient at a time, and only the two of them know what goes on between them. Those who are in training may occasionally be observed through one-way mirrors or have interviews taped for supervision, but as they become experienced enough to be considered capable of independent work, many become increasingly reluctant to expose details of what they say and do to colleagues who might criticize or ridicule their technique. A few brave ones, like the well-known psychoanalyst Merton Gill, have been willing to make tape-recorded interviews and verbatim transcriptions available for research, but usually, the more prestige a therapist has, the more sensitive he or she becomes to public scrutiny. I have heard one famous psychoanalyst quoted as saying that he might be willing to make such material available if he could be sure it would not be published until ten years after his death.

I know that when I myself re-read some of the comments I made in *My Language Is Me,* I wince and cringe and wonder why anyone ever sent me another patient after its publication. I felt that way even when I first discussed the material with Dr. Fromm-Reichmann, and I doubt that I would ever have let anyone else see it if she had not taken pains to convince me that the value of such material lies precisely in showing the mistakes, the tentative approaches, and the ordinary human frailties that show up in every psychotherapeutic relationship, along with the interventions about which the therapist may have reason to feel satisfied. I guess I was willing to risk it because I felt that what the boy was doing was so interesting, and because the case actually came out pretty well. In any event, at that time I didn't have all that much prestige to lose, and quite a bit to gain from writing a book if it turned out to be successful.

Another reason verbatim material seldom gets published is that it is hard to collect and still harder to put into readable form once it has been collected. Some types of patients, including the boy I wrote about, could not be tape-recorded without destroying his already fragile ability to trust anyone. Remembering exact interchanges in sequence after an interview is difficult and subject to distortion, and the attempt to fix details during an interview may interfere with the free floating attention that is most desirable in the therapist.

It just so happened that throughout most of his therapy, my patient tended to bring up one fairly well-defined topic after another, with long pauses in between, so that I could tick off the topics on my fingers and have time to remember what we had both said without seriously impeding my ability to listen. Immediately after each interview, I jotted down the topics, which seldom numbered more than ten, and then filled in the words each of us had said while they were still fresh in my mind. This meant that I had to rearrange my schedule to leave sufficient time before the next patient. It also inevitably created some counter-reactivity to the patient on my part, which might have led to problems but did not happen to damage the therapy significantly. I recognized, as did everyone else, that this kind of recording can never be completely accurate, but it was as accurate as I could make it, even when I had to record some remark of mine that I regretted immediately after making it. This took a great deal of restraint and soul-searching on my part, but I made a strenuous effort not to cheat.

Even when a therapist feels comfortable in tape-recording an interview, there are usually difficulties in writing the material up. I'm sure there exist many thousands of taped interviews in psychotherapy and analysis, but the very volume of words and the vast expenditure of time needed to go over them causes them to lie mouldering in file cabinets and storerooms. A busy clinician has to be especially motivated to collect and write up the material on a whole case.

Finally, this kind of material is hard to get published because of the difficult problem of maintaining confidentiality. This is particularly acute when case material is made available to the general public rather than appearing only in scientific publications with little circulation outside the profession. Even when the material has been carefully disguised to protect a patient's identity and he or she has granted permission to have it printed, a book may be read by friends and relatives of the patient who may recognize who it is about if for no other reason than that they know the person was treated by that particular therapist, and may penetrate the disguise. I'll give you an example of difficulty in maintaining confidentiality from the publication of *My Language Is Me.*

When I finally decided that I really did want to make a book out of it, the patient was twenty-two years old and near the end of his treatment. He was fully competent to discuss in detail his feelings about being written up as a case study, and by the time we were through discussing it, felt quite positive about making a contribution to knowledge that might help some other young person with problems similar to his own. He readily signed the release required for publication, I disguised the material carefully to protect his anonymity, and the book was accepted. It had been edited and was already in page proof before someone raised the question of whether we needed a release from the parents because the boy had been a minor at the beginning of treatment.

By the time a book has reaches the stage of page proof, the publisher already has a big financial investment in it, and the author has to pay if even a comma is changed. In order to project the boy's privacy, I was unwilling to ask for a release from the parents because in order to do so I would have had to admit to them that the book was about their son. I knew that if they saw the book they might suspect, but I also knew that they knew I had many other adolescent patients with similar problems, and they never could be really sure which one I was writing about. I assured the publisher of this, but he was unwilling to go ahead without a release for fear that at some point the parents might feel that their privacy had been invaded and might sue us all. We were stalemated, and I'm sure the book would never have been published if the publisher hadn't already invested so much in it.

We finally compromised: I rewrote certain sections in which the boy had discussed his views of his parents' problems, and the publisher and I agreed to split the cost of the revisions. Actually, this decreased the value of the material, because the parents and their problems were important factors in the boy's life. Many people afterward complained to me that the parents were too "shadowy." But it had to be done. Since we had a publication deadline in the near future, I sat up day and most of the night for three days, the to-be-deleted text on a triple-spaced sheet before me, typing the revisions under each line so that they would fill exactly the same space down to the last punctuation mark. I can tell you that I sweat blood until that book was finally off the presses! If, at that point, it hadn't gotten published, I would have died of a broken heart. But there was no way I could violate the trust of that boy by revealing his identity to his parents. Today, in the increasingly litigious climate of the United States, I doubt that any publisher would take such risk.

It is easier to avoid such problems if one writes novels. In a scientific treatise which is read largely by professional readers, you can omit so much and make descriptions so impersonal that nobody can be offended. In my kind of books, however, I tried to do the nearly impossible, although I didn't realize it until afterward. I clearly stated that the books were not fiction, but tried to write scientifically accurate material in such a non-technical and dramatized style that anyone interested in mental illness, layman or professional, could understand them and read them as though they were novels interspersed with comments by the author.

I had originally intended them for a primarily professional audience, not necessarily only psychiatrists, but non-medical therapists, counselors, and school personnel who might be dealing with similar young people. In a way it was both my luck and my misfortune that the publishers thought these books had potential appeal to the general public, and marketed them with that in mind. This was particularly true of *A Mingled Yarn*.

In order to make the book as successful as possible, the press did everything in its power to arrange for wide publicity. This I appreciated very much, and I participated with considerable excitement in all that was involved—reviews and interviews by major newspapers, television and radio appearances, and talks to groups all over the country. It scared me in a way, because I never felt quite prepared for what questions might be asked and at the time was not emotionally ready to acknowledge that the book was about my own family. However, it was a thrill to think of it as a potential best-seller, and I wanted to cooperate as well as I could. Unfortunately, the book seemed to fall between two markets, and nobody knew quite where it belonged. Booksellers whom I knew asked me whether to place it in the sections on fiction or psychology, and I would optimistically answer "Both!" Most booksellers didn't have a chance to ask me. (One of my friends, browsing in the book department of a large department store, found it in the knitting section.)

In spite of this, the books were fantastically successful by my standards. Both of them reached the audiences for which they were intended, as well as a lot of other people, were translated into German, and even made me a modest sum of money (although nobody in his or her right mind expects to get rich on a professional book unless it is a how-to book, a textbook, or a classic.) *My Language Is Me* was the Basic Book Club main selection for June 1962, went into several editions of popular paperback (Ballantine Books), and after being out of print in hardback for a number of years, is being re-issued by the Da Capo Press. *A Mingled Yarn* went into one edition of popular paperback (Fawcett) and then was published as a "quality paperback" by Yale University Press. I understand that now, nearly fifteen years later, they are well satisfied by its sale, but at the time people at the press were disappointed that it had not sold more widely, and so were the people, at Fawcett, for whom sales of less than half a million copies are not worth talking about. I'm sorry about that. I, too, would have liked to see it become a best-seller, but I never promised them a rosegarden.

In the spring of 1983, in the old Commodore Hotel in New York (which is now a Hyatt or a Hilton, or some such thing), I sat at a table on a dais in a ballroom and received the Frieda Fromm-Reichmann Award, given annually since her death by the Academy of Psychoanalysis for "Distinguished Contribution to the Understanding and Psychotherapy of Schizophrenia."

Receiving this award meant more than an honor to me. To me this award was a tribute to the person who first gave me the courage to write about my professional experiences in a way that made a difference and contributed immeasurably to my personal as well as my professional development. I only saw that person twice in my life and never really knew her, but as I rose to receive an award in her name, I felt that I stood there as a proxy for the one who started it all for me.

On Being a Woman
in a "Man's Profession"

The Uncle Toms of medicine— that's what radical feminists of today call women doctors of my generation, and they have a point. We entered the system in an era when most university medical schools, particularly the Ivy League schools of the East, had fairly recently and somewhat grudgingly begun to admit small quotas of women (Harvard had not yet accepted any), and we considered ourselves lucky to be among the chosen few. We were not about to rock a boat that held us quite precariously. If we didn't know it before we came to medical school, we knew soon afterward that many, if not most, of the men, both faculty and students, looked upon us as queer fish for wanting to be there at all and that if we wanted to be accepted as individuals, we had to do good work and see to it that our behavior was professional to the nth degree. We made every effort to fit into the system without trying to alter it and neither expected nor received any concessions to our femininity.

If any individual discriminated against us while we were students I was unaware of it. I never saw a member of the faculty treat any woman unfairly, rudely, or even in the slightest degree informally. The lab assistants and young instructors horsed around and made jokes with the boys, but not with us. Everyone was, in fact, almost unnaturally polite. No snide remarks were made within the range of my hearing; nothing pornographic or overtly sexual; no personal comments of any kind. It was almost as though we were invisible except as a vague, purifying force, and we did our best to keep it that way.

Relationships with our fellow students were equally benign. Most of them were friendly, treated us as peers, and worked with us on a level of equality, neither sparing us the unpleasant jobs nor shoving them upon us. Even though I was seven years older than most of my classmates, and I am sure was considered a little standoffish by some, I made a few good friends among them. Three women in our class later married classmates although to my knowledge there was little sexual fraternizing while we were in school. The women tried to walk a thin line—to be accepted as one of the boys without going so far as to be considered masculine. To be in the remotest degree seductive with anyone was an absolute no-no. In this manner we all got along quite well.

Yet the women as a group were never fully integrated into student life. As I mentioned earlier, they were segregated in the dormitory, and neither the men nor the women were allowed anywhere near each other's living quarters even for informal socializing. I don't know whether the men kept files of former exam questions, as I have heard they did in many medical schools, but if so nobody offered to share them with us. In the dining room the women sat together, not because they preferred each other's company, but because that had always been the custom. During my four years in that dormitory, only one woman persistently sat at one of the men's tables. So far as I know, none of the men objected. However, since that particular young woman segregated herself from the other women almost totally, we women looked upon her with the slight scorn which is so often the product of envy, and nobody else attempted to emulate her. Not even our best friends among the men ever invited any of us to do so.

In other words, discrimination took place not through the actions of individuals but through the structure and customs inherent in the system—the old boy networks, the student fraternities, the exclusion of women from the informal camaraderie and informal social life of their classmates except when small groups went together after class for a beer at the local bar and grill.

I have mentioned before that at P & S competitiveness among students was both assumed and encouraged. Between the women, however, this was not an issue; our only concern was to avoid being weeded out. We helped each other, studied for exams together, and we all sincerely hoped that none of us would fall by the wayside. We were not competing with the men either; we were trying to stay alive. Most of us hovered at or near the middle of the class, where we could be comfortably tolerated by the men who also did not seem to be competing against us. However, I have no doubt at all that had any of us been outstanding students reaching for top honors, the picture would have been very different. That's where the real competition took place.

The only male classmate from whom I encountered direct hostility was one of the top men in the class who, fearful that I might get a better grade than he because on one rare occasion the professor complimented me in public for making a difficult diagnosis, later "jokingly" accused me of using my feminine wiles to curry favor—me, who hadn't dared even to smile at the professor. It was true in those days, and I am reasonably sure it is still true, that many men can tolerate the success of female colleagues well only when they feel no threat of being overshadowed. When that threat appears, they may protect their egos by reverting to the use of stereotypes.

I have already made it clear that my experience as a woman doctor after the United States entered World War II was not typical of what most women experienced either before that era or afterward. The country needed our services, few men were available for civilian positions, and women in general had unusual opportunities for advancement. I don't know how many women today become chief residents at first-class university hospitals, but the fact that Babies Hospital in New York, part of the prestigious Columbia-Presbyterian Medical Center, had two of them within the two years between 1943 and 1945 would have been unimaginable a few years earlier. That I, who had had a mediocre record in medical school, could have become chief resident on the pediatric service of the University of California Hospital in San Francisco would have been considered even more bizarre. Now that the percentage of women in medical schools has risen so dramatically, perhaps women will again have access to such positions, but from what I hear and read, it is still quite unusual to find them there although there are always a few who manage to break through the barriers. Those few are apt to be unusually determined and talented people.

For some years before the time of my internship at Babies Hospital many of the faculty doctors had been women, some of them, like Hattie Alexander and Dorothy Anderson, famous in the field of pediatrics for their pioneering research on diseases of infants and children. All of them were well liked by the hospital personnel. They were respected by everyone, and their authority was unquestioned. For a number of years, there had also been a fair proportion of women among the interns, and nurses were accustomed to accepting them without friction. However, the majority of faculty and trainees had always been men, and the preponderance of women throughout the hospital staff during the war years brought on problems between the interns and nursing staff that nobody had anticipated.

Most of the head and assistant head nurses on the six patient floors were unmarried women in their late twenties and thirties who had been in charge of their wards for a number of years. In addition to being well trained and experienced in handling care of the children, they were competent teachers and secure in their role as administrators. They showed loyalty and often personal affection for the attending physicians on their wards, who, in turn, treated them respectfully, showing their appreciation for the heavy responsibility the nurses were carrying. However, at that moment in history, the nurses had a problem they found hard to cope with. Until that time all new interns, both male and female, had had at least a year of experience in some other hospital, but now suddenly over half of us were right out of school, and all but three of us were women.

Those young nurses were human, and for the most part they very much missed having men around the wards. Not only were they more accustomed to accepting the authority of male doctors, even young ones, but they had enjoyed the bantering, often sexually tinged, and playful relationships that are common between interns and nurses and the off-duty socializing that is such an important part of every young person's life. Suddenly they were faced with the loss of all that plus the responsibility of working with a group of authority figures most of whom were around their own age and far less knowledgeable then they about running a ward and caring for patients. Most of these authority figures were young women who were as frustrated by the lack of male companionship as they themselves were. The atmosphere in which we all worked during those years was highly charged.

It is dangerous to generalize about a whole professional group such as nurses because personalities and attitudes of individuals within the group vary enormously. But I think it would be safe to say that beneath the surface of compliance forced upon them by their training, a good many nurses carry a burden of resentment about their subordination to doctors, particularly to young doctors who, in the eyes of the nurses, have not yet achieved the status of good father or mother figures. I think it is also safe to say that a good many nurses also feel considerable competitiveness and envy toward doctors and that these feelings are more apt to be stirred up by doctors of their own age and sex. Individual nurses are not always aware of such feelings, but when stress situations weaken their defenses, the feelings may be expressed in various subtle and not so subtle ways which make for difficulty between people who are trying to carry out their separate roles to reach a common goal.

Inexperienced doctors have their own problems coping with feelings about subordinates who obviously know a lot more about what the doctors should be doing than the doctors themselves know. The need to protect an often inflated sense of their own importance may make them act in peculiar ways. Some handle their insecurity by becoming very authoritarian and throwing their weight around; others overcompensate for feelings of superiority by acting excessively meek and indecisive. It is difficult for both nurses and doctors under stress conditions to hit just the right balance in a relationship where the doctor must maintain authority without making the nurse feel put down and the nurse must demonstrate her superior knowledge about many things without putting the doctor down. On the basis of long tradition, it is often easier to accomplish this when the doctor is male.

Most of the female interns at Babies tried very hard to be friendly and egalitarian with the nurses, showing willingnesss to learn from them without overdoing a display of humility. It wasn't always easy, however, especially when some of the nurses consistently went over our heads to the older doctors for instructions or re wrote our orders without consulting us. When the chips were down, it was the intern's responsibility to plan and supervise the patients' treatment, and the intern was held accountable for incorrect orders. Attempts to protest having their authority subverted often led to open warfare in which the interns were not always successful.

Everyone knew that the head nurse on one of the wards was carrying on a long-term affair with the attending physician and felt secure in running the ward her own way regardless of orders or lack of them. An older nurse who presided over the ward for private patients considered interns as young puppies romping around under her feet—cute but totally inconsequential. She had known most of the private doctors for many years, dealt directly with them in spite of rules to the contrary, and absolutely ignored any orders written by the interns. In both of these cases no intern made the slightest attempt to protest; we tried only to remain on good terms with the nurses and stay out of their way. In other cases, however, individuals whose authority had been challenged clashed violently with one nurse or another. I remember one occasion when I myself became so angry with a nurse that I very nearly got into a hair-pulling brawl with her in the middle of the ward on morning rounds. Such incidents didn't occur often, but the potential was there and it created a lot of tension.

Most of the time we managed to get along together, which was lucky for us. An intern can be saved from a thousand disasters by the co-operation of a good nurse, and can be sabotaged in a thousand big and small ways by one who is antagonistic. In retrospect I consider it little short of a miracle that all the women in both professions came through those two years of manpower shortage with pretty good feelings about each other, and I think the efforts of both doctors and nurses can take credit for that.

Women doctors have always had, and to some extent continue to have, a handicap because, although it is gradually lessening, prejudice against them still pervades the population. Many people, particularly men, hesitate to consult them professionally, and they may be accepted ambivalently not only by some women but by their own male colleagues. However, well-trained and competent women have always been able to compete successfully with men in all the specialties they have entered.

Until the present time, certain medical specialties have been considered most suitable for women, particularly pediatrics, psychiatry, and public health. Women have been encouraged to enter these field presumably because their maternal qualities would be an asset but also, I am sorry to say, because these particular specialties have a lower income potential than some others like surgery or internal medicine and are less attractive to many of their male counterparts. Women have gone into them not because they feel themselves to be temperamentally more suitable or because they are resigned to making less money than men, but at least in part because public health and psychiatry offer opportunities for part-time work and greater schedule flexibility. this feature appeals to many women, especially those with small children or other family responsibilities.

Although nurturant impulses may have something to do with bringing both men and women into pediatrics, many doctors of both sexes leave that field after a while to enter psychiatry or public health. The Commonwealth Fund gave up offering training in psychiatry to pediatricians because after finishing their fellowships so many of the pediatricians became psychiatrists. In my years of teaching at the school of public health, a high percentage of all my classes was composed of ex-pediatricians entering the maternal and child health program.

The concentration of women in these three branches of medicine is one thing that is changing rapidly, and it is reasonable to expect that quite a number of women will soon be seen in all medical specialties, including surgery. Many are already preparing for careers in obstetrics and gynecology. Ironically, this is partly due to the fact that many women are now stereotyping women as they have always been stereotyped by men, feeling that females are bound to be more sensitive to the physical and emotional aspects of pregnancy and woman's disease than they think men are. This same feeling about womens' greater sensitivity has increased the demand among feminist women for female doctors, just as there was a demand for female doctors around the end of the nineteenth century when men didn't want other men to see their wives unclothed. (At that time, 6 percent of the total number of doctors were women, a percentage which decreased markedly after 1900 and was not equalled again until after the 1950s.)

In my profession I have met no discrimination on the basis of being a woman, but I have never sought high office in professional politics or high academic rank in medical school. I taught a graduate course in the School of Public Health at U.C. for many years, and both taught and supervised in the S.F. medical school department of psychiatry. In both places I chose to be titled lecturer, remaining off the academic ladder toward clinical professor. Politically or academically ambitious women had an uphill struggle in the past, and many still do.

At one time, many years ago, the nominating committee of a local psychiatric society asked me to run against another woman for president of the organization, saying "We think it's about time we had a woman." I refused, saying that I preferred not to be their token woman, and would run only against a man whom I considered a worthy opponent. I did, and lost in a perfectly fair competition. A woman had founded that organization, and was its first president, but until recent years no other was even nominated, although quite a few were elected secretary. In spite of the relatively high percentage of women in the membership of the American Psychiatric Association, a woman president was elected for the first time in 1985. These are only a few of the countless examples to show that males still dominate politically even in a field where many women successfully practice the profession.

None of the women doctors with whom I trained or whom I knew as colleagues throughout my years of practice have taken any part in organizations specifically for women doctors. We wanted to be accepted among our professional peer group as doctors, not as women doctors. None of us, I am sorry to say, were thinking in terms of benefiting other women by our participation. In retrospect, I think this was a rather arrogant attitude, and if I had it to do over again, I would join despite my reluctance to participate actively in any kind of organization. However, I cannot see that such organizations have had much influence in speeding up the acceptance of women into true professional equality. Things are changing, but as yet the changes have not been as great as one would like to hope.

Women doctors, more than men, have a problem that must be handled one way or another. This is the problem of their feelings about being envied by other women. They are envied, whether they like it or not or whether they recognize it or not.

I think it safe to say that in our culture, almost everyone envies the prestige and power wielded by highly paid professionals and corporate executives of both sexes. Doctors in particular have an awesome image not only because they are seen as rich and powerful, but also because they are seen as humanitarians who gain great intangible rewards in satisfaction from their work as well. This image is slipping at the present time, and is in many cases quite disproportionate to the actual facts, but the very title "M.D." has an almost magical effect upon a large number of people.

Envy is an emotion which automatically causes mixed feelings toward its object—admiration mixed with resentment which may remain unconscious when positive feelings predominate. To envy is considered a sin by some people; by others it is considered unworthy, making the envier feel humiliated and guilty. It is hard on both the one who envies and the one who is envied, arousing in both parties various kinds of internal defenses against recognizing the feeling as well as causing reactive behavior toward each other.

Being envied may be particularly hard on women doctors who want to be friends with women outside their own profession and have to confront evience of other women's ambivalence toward them. Even women who are perfectly contented with their own lives and haven't the slightest inclination to do the work of a doctor tend to feel some envy toward someone of their own sex who has the status of an M.D. This is particularly true of women in professions allied with medicine— nurses, social workers, or psychologists whose prestige is almost always less than that of the doctor even when the importance of their work is comparable or better than his or hers. A great many of them, along with teachers, particularly college teachers whose level of education is as high or higher than that of the doctor but far less adequately compensated financially, quite openly admit feeling competitive with and envious of doctors. Those who are not able to admit this to themselves and others nevertheless give many subtle evidences of their ambivalent feelings, which may be painful to the doctors who allow themselves to be aware of their own feelings.

Some people, of course, get gratification from being envied, but many people do not, especially if being envied is connected in their minds with traumatic experiences in earlier life, as was the case with me. In both instances they may need to protect themselves by not perceiving the evidence of envy directed toward them in close relationships. This is sometimes a handicap to psychotherapists, male or female, and for all doctors who have friends outside their own profession it may create perplexing misunderstandings.

Two of my closest personal friends were psychiatric social workers, and the public health nurse with whom I worked in the well-baby clinic remained for thirty years, one of my best friends outside the medical profession. All of them were happily married women, secure financially and interested in their own work. In each case we cared for each other and shared much of our lives, both professional and social yet all of them at one time or another gave evidence of ambivalence toward me which really hurt. All of them, when confronted, admitted that their underlying envy of me for having an M.D. was responsible for some resentment which they had not recognized until I brought it to their attention.

I do not generalize from a few cases. Over the years I have dealt with hundreds of women in various capacities—as patients, students, consultees, wives of colleagues, and other personal friends both those who are active in other professions and non-professionals engaged in many kinds of interesting artistic and volunteer activities. I have heard their envy of women doctors acknowledged by many, and perceived evidence of it from most. I believe it to be practically universal in our culture. Women doctors need to recognize it and learn to deal with the problem.

All women who enter "a man's profession," or aspire to levels of business hitherto reached only by men, have to face and live with one other entrenched attitude that is prevalent in our society. It would be charitable to think that when my friend who was applying for medical school back in the 1930s was asked why she thought only second-rate women wanted to enter medicine, the interviewer meant only to test her reaction to unexpected attack. Not entirely true, however. Whatever other reason he may have had, that doctor was expressing an attitude prevalent throughout not only the general population of the United States, but throughout the medical profession as well—an attitude that has not changed much in the fifty years since that time.

In what is probably a majority of men's minds, femininity by definition excludes a wish on the part of a woman to compete successfully with men in the marketplace. A woman in a "man's profession" is not quite a "real woman" in their eyes and in the eyes of a good many women as well. Any attempt by a professional woman to preserve her "feminine image" by dressing or behaving in ways that are traditionally considered feminine not only fails to dispel this attitude but instead opens the woman up to the image of an unfairly aggressive competitor trying to gain professional advantage by seducing her superiors—the old "feminine wiles" stereotype that I have already discussed. Ask any woman who has been advanced to a position of responsibility in a corporation whether at least one of her male colleagues has not "jokingly" accused her of sleeping with the boss. No wonder that the severe business suit and accompanying briefcase has become a uniform in which professional women are portrayed by TV and magazine ads today.

American culture as a whole, as well as members of the various professions and business communities, have accepted the idea that women can be first-rate doctors, architects, lawyers, and executives. It has not yet, however, accepted the idea that women in these formerly male professions can be considered first-rate in the realm of femininity. When people say to women professionals "You don't look like a doctor," they mean "You don't look like the stereotype of a de-sexualized woman." It is like when the British say "You don't seem like an American," meaning "You don't have a sharp nasal voice or act crass and insensitive." Everyone to whom that has been said knows that the speaker is unaware of how demeaning it is, and recognizes that it is intended as a compliment. Maybe young feminists of today will feel the need to make an issue of it, and maybe this will help change people's attitudes, but I really doubt it. I do know that women of my generation

simply tried to accept such remarks with good humor and learned to
live with the image.

On Working with Young People

When I go to professional meetings
these days, I locate my contemporaries by the white hair that stands
out here and there in the crowd. After forty years in the field, we are
the old-timers now—the former teachers of many younger colleagues
who are now taking our places just as we took the places of the professional generation that came before us. While many of our own teachers,
now approaching or into their eighties, are still wielding their influence,
many of them are already gone. We have become the top generation
in our profession—an awesome position to be in, and one that calls for
considerable humility in view of all the changes and problems con-
fronting the profession at this time in history.

I have been around a long time, and a lot of changes have already
taken place in the world around me, particularly in Berkeley, California—mecca for restless young people from all over the country who
seek an intellectually stimulating environment where innovative life
styles are acceptable. Over the years, I have witnessed the inner and
outer turmoil of numerous university student and faculty generations
during various eras of social unrest in which most of them were either
firm sympathizers or active participants in what was going on. Along
with them I have lived vicariously through disruptions caused by the
loyalty oath controversy of the late 1940s, the violence, rioting, and
rebellion of student sit-ins, Vietnam War protests and the People's
Park incident in the 1950s and 60s; the frustrated, passive protests of
the Haight-Ashbury flower children, the sexual freedom movements,
and the rising drug culture. I'm still around while members of the
present generation are getting arrested for non-violent protests against
nuclear power and the arms race. I have seen it all through many pairs
of eyes and have been involved in many conflicts of feeling, symptoms

produced by angers and anxieties, struggles to maintain any hope for the future of the world, and inner wars between idealism and cynicism.

Psychiatrists, of course, do not get a chance to work with people who are adjusting successfully to things the way they are in the world or with those who do not see themselves as needing help, even though, by our standards, they are often "sicker" than the ones who do. We talk mostly with troubled people. But among them are a good many thoughtful, sensitive ones—those whose discontents with what goes on in the world are not necessarily the result of personal neurosis or irrationality, although they may stir up degrees of anxiety unmanageable for all sorts of personal reasons. Our patients, along with a lot of other people, are not only struggling to handle the normal instinctual and interpersonal conflicts associated with the process of growing up and living but struggling within the complexity of a world realistically threatened with total extinction—a world realistically plagued by grave social injustice, overpopulation, mechanization, depersonalization, alienation, and other disruptive forces. Certainly no previous generations have been faced with such rapid changes in almost every aspect of society, nor, before television revolutionized communication in the 1950s, was there ever such widespread awareness among the young of what goes on in disparate segments of the world they live in.

I do not intend to make this a discussion of the problems of society or of the generation gap, but I would like to say that in working therapeutically with such people, I have had to work at keeping my mind open to new ideas and at realizing that the impact of those ideas on young people may not be the same as it is on me or others of my age who were brought up in a very different world. It is hard, sometimes, to remember that many of the values that people of my generation took or still take for granted as normal in our society are being seriously challenged today by people who are by no means abnormal in any psychiatric sense or even particularly unconventional, since the conventions themselves have changed so much and vary considerably in segments of even "normal" middle-class society.

At the same time, it is not always easy to keep a clear distinction betwen the rational reactions of some young people to the irrational world in which they live and the irrational reactions of others to that same world—reactions which they attribute to the evils of the external environment in order to deflect their own and other people's attention from sources within themselves that give rise to the angers and anxieties they are feeling. It is not an either-or proposition. The fact that some people rebel legitimately against social wrongs does not mean that they have no personal emotional difficulties, nor does it mean that neurotic and psychotic individuals are not rebelling against real social problems.

I have spent a good deal of my professional life working with disturbed young people, at first on the University of California Student Health Service, and later in private practice, where for a long time a sizable proportion of my patients were late adolescents between the ages of sixteen and thirty. Some people will immediately say thirty is too old to be put in this category, but Berkeley is a college town, where many members of that age group are still students who are both emotionally and financially tied to their parents. Here my old-fashioned ideas may be showing, but in my opinion, those who are called adult should, by definition, have worked through most of the adolescent conflicts over growing up and be more or less able to function independently. A thirty-year-old student often still identifies with the somewhat younger youth culture, and many of the sixteen-year-olds identify with the same values as their somewhat older peers. In any case, my patients have belonged to the youth culture.

I think perhaps after my return from New Haven I became type-cast as someone with a knack for working with this age group, especially after I published a book about working with a disturbed sixteen-year-old boy. From then on, for a number of years most of my referrals were young, middle-class, educated, and turbulent boys and girls, some merely relatively normal people in some kind of emotional crisis, but many in the diagnostic categories of schizophrenics who were not disorganized enough to require hospitalization and what we now call borderline personality disorders. It is not always easy to make a distinction between these categories, or even between the pathological and the relatively normal patients, because they may exhibit very similar behavior and share significant characteristics. Fortunately, my method of treating the individuals psychotherapeutically did not vary all that much, and I did not find that pinning an exact label on anyone was very useful.

In the last thirty-five years there have been great changes in the field of psychiatry, and a great number of therapeutic methods have been developed, all of which seem to work for some people and none of which works for everyone. There are over two hundred recognized types of psychotherapy, not to speak of all the other forms of therapy offered by both psychiatrists and non-medical therapists. I'm sure all this makes the insurance companies very unhappy, because it is hard to tell what to consider legitimate therapy, as well as what is effective for any particular condition or for any particular individual. The increasing use of therapeutic drugs has confused things even more, and within the field itself there are violent disagreements and controversies not only between different schools of thought but between individual therapists within each school.

I am not prepared to make a judgment on what is the best method for treating the kind of young person I describe. I can only describe what I have observed about them over the years and what I, with the particular training and personality I have, have found effective. The method I use is a relatively conservative but not inflexible form of analytically oriented psychotherapy, meaning that it is conducted within a framework of analytic principles, although it is by no means a mini-analysis.

Most of these patients, in spite of their individual differences, have certain characteristics in common. The first is a grossly defective sense of self-esteem. No matter how they present themselves, no matter how arrogant or on top of things they seem to be, most young people don't turn up in a crisis situation unless they have a very wobbly feeling about their own worth. Because self-esteem and the ability to love someone else go hand in hand, they frequently have real difficulty caring for another in a mature way. This is particularly striking at the present time. With the new sexual freedom, a lot of what passes for relatedness isn't that at all, and although the individuals may be able to function sexually, they are not functioning emotionally. They generally have poor impulse control, particularly control over aggressive impulses, low tolerance for frustration, and confusion about their sexual identity.

In the past fifteen years or so, relatively few young people with the type of pathology just described have come to me for the kind of therapy that I and most analysts practice. The ones who have were all in a rather special group. I cannot remember having had a turbulent late-adolescent patient since around 1960 who was not either the child of someone in one of the mental health professions or a young person who had had a close relationship with some adult who had previously been analyzed or successfully treated in some way by an analyst. What is more, all such patients who came to me have, in spite of great ambivalence, had enough trust in the referring adult to accept the possibility that this form of treatment would benefit them. It was usually this borrowed trust that enabled the patient to stay in treatment. Nowadays many young people in these diagnostic categories seem to be using some form of social protest to relieve their tension, are seeking the more action-oriented or supposedly direct therapies, or are turning to cults, mystical religions, or drugs. I believe this is to be expected from the nature of their pathology, which is dominated in most cases by intolerance for frustration and anxiety.

I can't speak about these other forms of therapy, because there are so many of them and because I have not really studied what the various ones accomplish. Of course, people in my situation see as patients only the failures, who come to us to be put together again after they have fallen apart. I may be biased, but I think what happens in a lot of these more active therapies is felt by patients as a head-on assault on their self-esteem. That is difficult to handle, and quite a few do come apart. I myself worked for a long time with a man who had been a pretty well put-together person in spite of numerous anxieties, but became psychotic during primal scream. He couldn't stand what the regression did to his self-esteem, and it took a long time for him to recover.

Along with the confusion that many of these young people feel about their maleness or femaleness, therapists often see what used to be called polymorphous perverse trends in sexual behavior. The tenor of the times makes it difficult to distinguish deep-seated pathology from sexual acting out, because nowadays it is very acceptable in certain youth groups to experiment with activities that used to be called perversions. One isn't supposed to call anything a perversion any more; anything done between consenting adults is permissible. I agree with that in principle, but often the behavior is not accompanied by any sense of real relationship, as I said before, and a good many of the young people with whom I have worked have had their anxieties greatly increased rather than decreased by this kind of "freedom." Some of them, who may not have really deep-seated thinking disturbances, tend to drift into more primitive forms of thinking and the kind of symbolic talk that I tried to demonstrate in *My Language Is Me.*

Even though a good many of the older members of these groups were referred to me for analysis, I see none of them in classical analysis. I believe most firmly that for them, and for most adolescents, analysis is not the treatment of choice. Some analysts disagree with me, but that's what I believe. Adolescents are still in a formative state where they need real adults to identify with, not the relatively anonymous analyst whose main activity concerns interpretation of the transference. I think it is important to operate from a framework within which people know exactly where the limits are; but most of these patients cannot stand the frustration of talking for long periods of time with almost no response from the therapist.

I also do not believe that all therapists can work with all patients. In my opinion, in order for successful work to take place, a kind of fit has to develop fairly soon; if it does not, it is better for everyone to refer the patient elsewhere. This is particularly true with younger patients. A fit can develop between the most unlikely personalities, but it has to develop, and for this reason, along with many others, a therapist has to be well aware of his or her own reactions as well as those of the patient.

Over the years, I have found very few patients I didn't come to like rather soon after starting to work with them, and when I did find one it was usually my problem, not the patient's. There are obviously quite a few unlikable people people in the world, but what makes a person likable to one may cause dislike in another according to his or her previous experience. I, for instance, tend to like people who are honest, direct, and outspoken about their feelings, even though such people are sometimes tactless and may have trouble getting along with their friends or employers. I tend to find very wearing those who go through life with bland optimism, using a euphemistic, sweetness and light approach, although such people may be quite popular with their peers. Although I recognize the source of my countertransference in the un-realistic optimism and sweet stubbornness of my own mother, the recognition does not always dispel the irritation I feel when I encounter these traits in others. There have been very few times when I can remember feeling persistent dislike of any patients after I came to know them and understand why they act the way they do, but if I couldn't overcome my own countertransference feelings, I have usually told them that I don't think we fit together, and they usually accept it, because by the time I have been ready to say it, they have already become aware of it. A few years ago I had such an experience with a sixteen-year-old girl, and she was aware of it before I was. That was the first time I really felt the generation gap, although I guess I will have to expect it more often from now on.

This girl, the daughter of two well-educated professional people, was rebelling against her conservative upbringing and had already slept with a large number of men. In the course of telling me about that, she used as exceedingly vulgar term for sexual intercourse—not the usual vernacular, but a term I had never before heard used by anyone except a particularly coarse man. I tried to point out to her that the use of that term was evidence of her depreciation of her own sexuality, but she just looked at me with a sneer and said, "You are too old for me. Everyone I know uses that term, and you just aren't hep to the lingo." Well, actually I am quite hep to the lingo, or at least was during that particular period, but I said to her, "I think you are right. I really feel too old for you, and I think we had better not try to work together." I knew that her attitude was a resistance to therapy, but at the same time, it was a resistance she could appreciate more easily if she worked with a younger therapist who could then point out other forms of it.

I occasionally do still work with adolescents, but I now find that the ones with whom I can empathize best are not the more overtly chaotic types but those whose feeling of chaos is more internalized. I have passed into a different stage in my own professional and personal development.

The private practice of psychiatry is a very fascinating business for psychotherapists, and they do go through different phases in their own professional development. At least I did, and so did most of the colleagues with whom I have discussed the matter. Those who are just starting out get a lot of their satisfaction just from seeing examples of the kinds of pathology they have been learning about in their training. In other words, the content of the material is of interest, and so are the personalities of the patients. In looking through my records on people I worked with for fewer than ten sessions, I can picture very clearly most of the early patients, although I remember little about their problems or the technical aspects of their therapy. Those who came later, sprinkled throughout the years, I cannot always picture, but I often remember quite a bit about the course of my work with them. Apparently the focus of my interest had shifted to working out technical problems. Of course I also remember the funny problems, like that of a man who wanted help in dealing with his mother-in-law. He was "happily married" but had been sleeping with his mother-in-law as well as his wife for many years; he now wanted to stop with the mother-in-law, but she was holding him by threatening to tell his wife about the relationship. The scary ones also tend to stick in my mind—

the avowed sadist who told me how he liked to throw live goldfish into boiling water to see them explode, or the young man who suddenly rose from the chair, leaned across my desk, and asked, "What would you do if I attacked you right now?" These kinds of situations are by no means the most interesting, but they do tend to be remembered.

From the time that I found it necessary to decide whom to treat from among referrals, I have chosen to work for the most part with those whose problems are amenable to long-term analytic exploration, whether in actual classical analysis or by modifications of the technique without the use of medication. This often requires a great deal of persistence on the part of the therapist and a strong motivation on the part of the patient. In the end, however, it is worth the effort that both put into it and rewarding to both. It remains to be seen whether the type of practice I have enjoyed will survive all the changes that are now taking place in the field, with insurance companies and other third-party payers calling the shots on what kinds of therapy they consider cost-effective. It will be sad if we revert to a situation where only the relatively well-to-do can have a kind of treatment which, although sometimes more expensive and certainly more time-consuming, may be the treatment of choice for a considerable number of people.

On the Conflicts of Professional Women Today

As I have gotten older, the nature of my practice has changed somewhat. Nowadays a good many of my patients seem to be middle-class, educated women in their late thirties and early forties who are either depressed about the way their lives have gone or in conflict over the way they want them to go. Many women, affected by the feminist movement, are confused by changes in the social and sexual roles now demanded of them and suffer at least partly as a result of problems related to social and sexual identity which confront them in today's social climate. While talking to these women, I have to stay constantly aware of the fact that many of my own attitudes were formed in another era, under quite different circumstances, and that I must be particularly careful not to impose them on my patients who face different social attitudes in the modern world.

The feminist movement has been immensely effective in making women aware of themselves as women and in making both men and women aware that many changes in attitude and custom are long overdue. I believe that the overall results have been, and will increasingly be, beneficial to the whole of society. But at the same time, a lot of conflicts have been created and a lot of anxiety stirred up in both sexes which many individuals find hard to handle.

I can't speak for the attitudes of all women throughout the United States as a whole. My only professional experience has been in psychologically sophisticated communities like New Haven and Berkeley, but I imagine the patients in these cities pretty well represent the population that most analysts and analytic psychotherapists see in their offices. These are middle- and upper-middle-class women with at least high school and more often college educations, many with graduate degrees. These are the ones who have sufficient motivation, insurance coverage, and/or private funds to seek help with such problems.

I think it likely that with patients of this kind in many such communities one would find self-assertive attitudes among women that are reflected in their approach to therapy. It has become extremely common for women wanting help with their conflicts to feel that men cannot possibly empathize with their feelings and to seek out women therapists, who they think will be more understanding. It is also quite common for these women to seek women therapists whom they consider sympathetic to feminist goals. Just what this means varies with individuals, but gone are the days when such patients just went compliantly to anyone to whom they had been referred, assuming that the therapist would probably be competent enough to help them with their problems. Many of them now interview a prospective therapist as thoroughly as they would interview a prospective employee.

Gone, also, are the days when even a "classical" analyst could be anything remotely resembling a blank screen, even if the analyst wanted to be (as most no longer do). Many patients have already researched the credentials and reputation of anyone to whom they have been referred before they even make the first appointment, and often they also know quite a bit about the therapist's private life. Berkeley is not a very large community, and many social networks are intertwined. All this foreknowledge may create complications in the treatment, and the need for a patient to seek it out may mean many different things in different cases, but nevertheless, in my opinion, it is a very healthy trend. I myself would not dream of putting my life in the hands of a doctor without knowing something about him or her. Unfortunately, the privilege of having that kind of choice was previously restricted to professional colleagues who had the opportunity to get inside information.

In any case, many women who have come to see me over the past ten years or so have come at least partly because they have heard something about me and see me as someone who had reasonable success in both marriage and career during a period when their own mothers were "just housewives." They want to work with someone who they feel has faced the problems they now confront, but they do not always realize that my problems, both internal and external, were faced in an era of entirely different social expectations.

Presumably the emancipation of women is intended to give them a choice of what they want from life, but in many cases the choice is fraught with conflict. There are now tremendous peer pressures upon college-educated women to have a professional or high administrative business career. Not to want one is considered to be almost a disgrace. At the same time, in the culture as a whole, such women are still expected to marry and have a family. Often there is great pressure from their parents, who still want grandchildren regardless of whatever else their children may accomplish.

Most educated young women with whom I have talked want a family eventually, but not all of them want a career. Those who would prefer to build their lives around their families and confine their outside activities to volunteer work in the traditional way are, however, very much on the defensive. They now have the same choice that we had a generation ago—conform to the expectations of peers and take a job or go apologetically against the mainstream. The difference is that peer group expectations are exactly opposite from what they were in our day.

For my generation, the expectations of peer group and parents were more or less the same in most cases. Being "only" a wife and mother was perfectly acceptable to almost everyone. Both peers and parents were critical of a girl who wasn't married before the end of her twenties, and they simply assumed that if married, she would want a family. There was no conflict with the culture in making that choice, but now there is. Many young women feel not only apologetic but actually ashamed about being so unambitious."

Those who want a career instead of a family meet no real opposition from their peer group, but they are apt to suffer from being considered "incomplete women," the newest euphemism for "frustrated spinster," no matter how much sexual activity she may indulge in. Even her peers covertly look down on a women who does not want a child. As I said earlier, many parents, even those who are themselves in professions or academic life, put great pressure on their daughters to furnish them with grandchildren and still regard a childless daughter as not quite an adult, no matter how high she has risen in the business or professional world. These attitudes on the part of peers and parents get across to a young woman in many subtle and not so subtle ways, often leaving her depressed and defensive under a surface attitude of defiance.

A great many young women today are caught up in a network of ambivalent feelings—the wish to be modern and function on a basis of equality with men in the marketplace, the wish to be regarded as "complete women" by parents or peers, and the fear of failing if they try to do both. Many of those who come to me are asking, either explicitly or implicitly, for a formula on how to combine a successful family life with a successful professional career. If I had such a formula, the line of women waiting for it would soon stretch from my office to San Jose. Every individual is different from every other in her needs and desires; infinite variables determine what will work for each one. So many women I have talked to seem to feel they should be able to have it all—the perfect husband, the perfect job, perfect children—without anything having to give way for anything else. Judging from the high divorce rate, a lot of them are not getting everything they want. There are a few who do, and as a matter of fact, there were a few even in my day and earlier, but usually those few have been in rather special situations.

An example that any woman might envy in any era is that of Millicent Carey McIntosh, who was already dean of Bryn Mawr College at the age of twenty-seven and later married Dr. Rustin McIntosh, the head of Babies Hospital during the era of its greatest prestige, in the 1940s and 1950s. She became headmistress of the Brearley School in New York and while there had five children, all of whom did well and grew up to be doctors or professors. When they were still fairly young, she became dean and later president of Barnard College. She seems to me the ultimate in role models for professional women who also want to be mothers. Let us examine for a moment the conditions under which she accomplished these miracles.

1. Her education was completed and her academic career well established before she married.

2. She married a man who was also well established in a highly prestigious and lucrative career which was completely non-competitive and unrelated to hers. This man, even fifty years ago, was dedicated to the ideal of equal opportunity for women in the marketplace, and he was also dedicated to the ideal of having men share equally in concern for the family. *no*

3. There were ~~do~~ demands on her to take part in any activities outside her job and her family in order to further her husband's career—no need to entertain clients, socialize with those who might further his promotion, or take part in conspicuous charitable events to enhance his prestige.

4. She could afford and was able to obtain excellent help in taking physical care of the children when small.

5. Her job was five blocks from her apartment, and her time schedule was flexible enough so that she could go home for lunch and drop in on her children periodically throughout the day. She did not have to miss seeing their first smiles, hearing their first words, playing with them, and reading them stories. She could enjoy raising her children without in any way sacrificing the needs of her job, and her children could enjoy her prestige without feeling that interest in her work came ahead of their needs. No child of the McIntosh family had problems like those of the five-year-old daughter of two busy doctors who was referred to me years ago because she had mutilated herself in frustrated competition with her parents' patients.

6. I know nothing about the sex life of this ideal couple, but I have to assume that it was satisfactory enough to keep them peacefully together for fifty years, into their middle eighties, leading an active and productive life together.

Show me another women in that particular combination of circumstances, and I will guarantee her both a successful marriage and a successful career.

Those who look to me as a role model would not have the same guarantee. In fact, I cannot serve as a role model for them because I did not have to face what I consider the most difficult problem that most of them will encounter. Although by my own standards I did manage to combine success in marriage with a successful career, the circumstances under which I did so might not seem ideal to everyone.

I too had established the foundations of my career firmly before marriage. However, I was physically unable to bear children. That was the biggest sorrow of my life, but so far as my career went, it was an advantage. I could not have raised small children at the same time that I was carrying heavy professional responsibilities, and I would not have wanted to because I believe that my children would have suffered from it, and so would I.

If I had had small children, I would have wanted to spend a great deal of time with them in their early years, and although I might have been able to carry on a part-time practice while they were in school, I think I would constantly have felt torn between their needs and those of my patients. Some women are able to handle such conflicts or might not actually feel them, but I know many who do and who suffer from them. I have seen friends of mine rush away from an important professional conference because of a call from the babysitter, or leave to someone else the job of taking a sick child to the hospital because at the moment they couldn't leave a sick patient. These are the kinds of choices professional women with children have to face quite often, and it isn't easy to make them.

One might wonder whether being raised by a nurse myself has caused me to overvalue mothers caring for their own children in the earliest years. I am sure this is true to some extent, although actually my own experience might just as easily have prejudiced me in the other direction. My nurse was the most stable influence in my early life, and I have talked to many people raised by nurses who feel the same way. In disturbed family situations, a surrogate mother may be a godsend. However, I have to keep in mind that the Nannies, Fräuleins, and Mademoiselles of my era were full-time caretakers who often stayed with a family for many years. They were of a different breed than the babysitters, au pair girls, and live-in college students who are the only kinds of helper available to most professional mothers today who can afford help.

Even if they can afford it, it is particularly hard for them to get the kind of help they need when the child is an infant and young toddler. There are excellent day care centers, of course, but in most communities there are not nearly enough of them. In Berkeley, for instance, in order to get into some of the most desirable nursery schools, a child has to be enrolled at or before birth, and even then must sometimes face a long waiting list. In the newspapers these days, we have all read about horrors that can occur in some of the less desirable ones, and it is often difficult for a parent to distinguish one kind from another ahead of time.

As described earlier, I have worked closely with personnel at nursery schools for the children of working mothers and know that in spite of the disadvantages, good early child educational institutions have great potential for giving young children valuable learning experiences. I hope that eventually in our country privately financed child care centers, similar to those furnished in all large industrial organizations of the socialist countries, will be a part of our corporate structures, and that more state and local tax funds will be available for good community child care centers. When that time arrives, if it ever does, working women will have fewer worries about what is happening to their children while they are working. However, I have seen enough tired, cranky children being returned to tired, cranky mothers at the end of a nine-hour day care program to feel that day-long mother-child separations during the child's early years aren't very good for either the child or the mother.

In a relatively normal family situation, a child is better off forming its first attitudes toward itself and others in a relationship with its own mother rather than with a series of transient or even somewhat more permanent mother's helpers. The mother is better off too if she is privileged to enjoy her child's infancy. Many mothers cannot afford that luxury, but for those who can, there is no doubt in my mind that it is better for everyone. As I said earlier, the person who carries out most of the child's bodily care in the first two years becomes a primary identification figure, and I believe that most mothers would really prefer to be that figure if they can.

This does not mean that a mother should spend all her time with a small child. All mothers need to get away from their children for periods during the day. Nor do I think that mothers are neglecting their children by turning them over to others while they work, although often their own parents give them a bad time about this. I believe that it *is* impossible to do two full-time jobs at the same time and do both of them well. I have seen many women manage to work out the problems satisfactorily, but I have also seen many ambitious women, eager to go high in a profession or in the corporate world, who, when confronted with a conflict between the needs of the child and the needs of the job, are often forced to choose the needs of the job and are consumed by guilt about the situation.

I myself never had to face that difficult choice. My family came ready-made as teenage boys beyond the need for bodily care and almost independent of the need for much attention from me. I was therefore free to pursue my career without interruption. But my freedom from responsibility was purchased at some cost to my relationship with the boys, even under very advantageous circumstances; freedom from responsibility for one's children always exacts some price from somebody.

Many books have been written about relationships between men and women in these modern times. I do not intend to write another but speak only of the kinds of problems that have come to my attention in working with patients. What I hear is that most wives with professions of their own find there are demands upon them which often conflict— demands not only from the needs of their children, but also from the needs of their husbands even when there are no small children in the picture.

Whether her husband wants it that way or not, in many cases his job at times demands that his wife play a certain role—as hostess to clients and colleagues, for instance, or as participant in various kinds of social and charitable events along with the wives of colleagues or superiors who may have a lot to say about whether her husband gets a promotion. If the demands of her own job preclude this kind of participation, his status among his colleagues may suffer, and sometimes even the job itself. Can she tolerate the guilt about that? Can he accept the situation without resentment? Especially in the years when both the man and the women are on the way up in their professions, this may become a very touchy issue.

I have heard the sneers of older faculty wives when the wives of young instructors don't assume their proper role. I myself was spared much of this kind of criticism: my husband was already at the top of the ladder, beyond the need for competition in a departmental rat race. Also I was lucky enough to have a good friend among the faculty wives who liked to stand in for me when I should have been presiding at departmental teas. Punk and I had made an agreement at the start that if it was ever important for him to have me preside at university functions, I would cancel my patients, put on a hat, and try to act like a lady. Once or twice, while he was acting dean, he did request it, and I rather enjoyed doing it, but such times were few and far between.

The needs of his job did not interfere with mine, nor mine with his. I seldom called upon him to accompany me to professional affairs, knowing that a husband from another profession may feel considerably more awkward in a gathering of his wife's professional colleagues than a professional wife feels among her husband's colleagues. He, like most lay people, felt somewhat intimidated by psychiatrists and analysts in the mass, but he didn't feel his personal security threatened, and when I needed him, he came with good grace. Not every young women is in that happy position.

An increasing number of young couples in which both husband and wife have high-paying, well-established professions are finding themselves in a crisis when one person's opportunities for advancement require moving to another area. Will the wife abandon a good legal practice, for instance, so that her husband can accept a medical professorship in another part of the country? What will happen to their relationship if she considers her job as important as his and refuses to move? What if he considers his job more important than hers and insists on moving? How are they going to resolve this dilemma without destroying the marriage? I have seen a number of couples wrestle with such a problem, and it sometimes does destroy the marriage, although more often, I have to admit, the woman gives in and swallows her resentment. In spite of Women's Lib, that is still expected of her.

In the past, there would have been no question about whose job took precedence. The husband's job, of course, particularly since a generation ago few women had jobs as good as or better than their husbands'. Back in the 1960s, even after the boys were out of the home, if I had been offered a well-paying, high academic position in a department of psychiatry in the East, I would not even have considered it. It would have been out of the question, not only because neither of us wanted to leave our home, but because it would have been out of the question for me to ask Punk to give up his job at the university even though my job might pay better than his and he had transportable skills as a landscape architect. If he had felt it was important to me, he might have agreed, and nobody would have criticized him. For a man of his status to make such a sacrifice for his wife would have been considered noble and rather macho, but a wife who accepted such a sacrifice would have been considered a "castrating bitch" by everyone, including herself.

Things may be a lot different today in some circles, but I doubt it. A woman who asks her husband to sacrifice his career for hers is still considered a castrating bitch, even if the husband is willing. Most men can afford to be non-competitive with their wives only if they are themselves secure enough, both personally and in the status of their work.

Nowadays many young married (or unmarried and living together) couples who are both professionals or business executives are doing a wonderful job of sharing responsibility for housework and child care. This is no longer considered women's work in sophisticated circles where both men and women believe in equality of opportunity. Lots of men have not only learned to cook—they love to cook and do it as well as if not better than their wives. They are conscientious about sharing the drudgery—vacuuming, dusting, and bedmaking as well as taking out the garbage and other such jobs with which good husbands have always helped their wives. But this kind of mutuality often has an emotional cost.

Most men today who are in their thirties and forties have not been brought up for the domestic role they are trying to assume. Being a good husband hasn't been built into their psyches from the day they were born, and although they accept it intellectually, the deep-down emotional response doesn't always fit what they believe.

Perhaps by the time another generation rolls around, men will have been trained for the role of husband as women have traditionally been trained for the role of wife. The young women who are today the mothers of boys will have to see to that. Perhaps then men and women will have equal skills for all the roles required in their daily lives, and perhaps then a man's sense of masculinity and a woman's sense of femininity will not be threatened by the changes in social roles. In many cases it hasn't happened yet, however.

Regardless of their husbands' good intentions, many professional women find that they still have to assume major responsibility for running the household. Unless they can afford full-time help or can afford to eat out a good deal of the time, two tired people come home at the end of the day and both of them want to be nurtured. I have in mind two high-level young business executives who often don't get home until after eight o'clock at night. Although they usually go out to dinner, the husband resents the fact that he can't relax at home with a dinner waiting. When they do eat at home, the dinner is usually fast food or pizza, and it just isn't what his Mommy brought him up to expect. In a good many cases, the humdrum, ordinary, day-to-day scraping together of a simple dinner falls on the wife, who is just as tired as he is and resents having to be the one who does it, but recognizes his need as greater than her own. Sometimes she feels guilty about her resentment and sometimes not, but in both cases the resentment comes out in some other way.

I am very old-fashioned, but in my opinion, every household needs someone with major responsibility for keeping it running smoothly. Complete equality in assuming that responsibility is a noble ideal, but I'll be very much surprised if it turns out to be practical in the long run. Maybe eventually all families with two full-time breadwinners will be able to afford and to find good housekeepers, but it seems very unlikely.

When women ask me how they can combine a successful marriage with a successful career, I suggest that first of all they define what they mean by success in marriage. What can they tolerate, and what can they not? This is a very individual matter. For instance, I consider that Punk and I had a successful marriage, but to a lot of women it might not seem so. He and I were very different in some ways. We often spent fairly long periods together without verbal communication, when we were both preoccupied with quite different matters. This did not interfere with our basic sense of togetherness, but for couples who need constant verbal communication and stimulation from each other, it might be intolerable. There is no way that anyone can give advice without understanding the other person's needs and value system.

My own opinion is that the most important work a woman can do is raise healthy, productive, and reasonably happy children. I feel that if pursuit of a career conflicts with family needs, the family needs should have first priority. Some may consider this a very old-fashioned view, and I do not try to impose it on my patients, but that is what I think.

For women who want and are able to have children along with a career, I would say get your career established before you try to have a family. This in itself creates problems, as we see in many cases today where women in their late thirties and early forties, finally ready to have children, suddenly become aware that the biological clock may have stopped for them. However, if they don't just think they ought to want children in order to be considered a complete woman, and if they find they are able to have healthy ones; if they are willing to give up a lot of the freedom to which they have become accustomed *and* if their husbands feel the same way, I would say take a few years off during the early lives of your children and resume your career afterward, or work out some kind of part-time arrangement, or settle for a less ambitious position in the professional world where you can arrange for time off when you need it. If you can't do that, reconcile yourself to the fact that baby sitters and day care teachers will become primary figures of identification for your children.

Secondly, I would say try to find a man whose masculinity is not threatened by having a successful wife, preferably a man in another business or profession who will not be directly competitive with you. This should be easy in these days of enlightenment, but the millennium is not yet here.

I can cite the case of a couple I know who are both psychoanalysts, very enlightened. In the early days of their career, both applied for training in the psychoanalytic institute of a city where both wanted to live and had established good practices. Only the wife was accepted, so in order to preserve the marriage, they moved to another city where both were accepted to the same institute. Both were terribly unhappy about it, and his male ego was badly bruised in spite of his overt acceptance of the situation. The marriage survived, but the relationship between them was never the same again.

Lastly, and fervently I would say to these women, "Don't demand perfection, either in the job or in the marriage! If you haven't got the willingness or the capacity to compromise, don't try it, because unless you are one in a million, you aren't going to be able to have it all."

On Psychoanalysis

I had heard little about psychoanalysis until I was already a psychiatrist, in the mid-1940s, and did not think seriously about endering the field myself until I had spent some time in a training analysis undertaken purely out of desire for a therapeutic analysis with a particular analyst, Erik Erikson. This ignorance was due in part to the fact that I had come from a conservative segment of society, where radically new ideas were slow to be accepted, and in part to my somewhat neurotic self-preoccupation during the years of my college and early professional education. However, it was also due to the fact that psychoanalysis as a field of medical practice was just beginning to be established in the United States during the 1920s and 1930s, when I was growing up. Freud's ideas were at first little known in this country except within small circle of avant-garde intellectuals and academics and had not permeated the general culture as they did in the next two decades.

During the early 1930s, when I was in college, most educated people had heard about Freud, and some had read his works, but a great many had only heard his ideas derided and denigrated, as they still are by many people today. I cannot think whether this was the case with me, but I think it must have been. I do remember that in 1928, at the age of sixteen, while spending a boring summer in Los Angeles with my grandparents, I happened to find a copy of Freud's *Interpretation of Dreams* in the bookcase. This could only have been put there by my maiden aunt Helen, who had died earlier that summer after living most of her life with her parents. It could not possibly have been either brought there or read by my grandparents, who, although intelligent people, had not gone beyond high school in the 1860s, and could by no stretch of the imagination have been called intellectuals. As a matter of fact, neither could my aunt, whose education ended with finishing school in the 1890s.

My aunt, however, was deeply interested and well read in matters related to the occult, and Freud lay on that shelf nestled between books about astrology and chiromancy. I found tham all somewhat intriguing and browsed through all of them, but in my mind *The Interpretation of Dreams* was in the same category as the others—not worthy of being taken seriously. If I had read it then, I doubt that it would have made any sense to me. Although I cannot really remember now, I believe that I, along with most of the people I knew, thought of Freud as a weirdo in the same class as Coué, who was then the rage. ("Every day in every way, I'm getting better and better.") Nobody disabused me of this idea in college, perhaps because the courses I took were not in fields concerned with intellectual movements or theories of psychology.

It seems odd to me now that I didn't hear more about psychoanalysis in medical school and subsequent professional training, but analytic concepts were not routinely introduced into medical or even psychiatric education until the 1940s. In any case, psychoanalysis as a form of therapy was not mentioned during the course in psychiatry that I took as late as 1941. This seems particularly odd to me since one of our professors was Dr. Nolan C. Lewis, one of those who had shown an early interest in Freud's ideas, and my section instructor was Janet Rioch, a prominent New York analyst. Babies Hospital had an analyst on the staff—Hilda Bruch, who later became famous for her work on eating disorders—but although the house staff participated in her re-search on obesity in children, we did not think of her as an analyst, nor did she advertise herself as such. She impressed us with her ideas about the kinds of family structures and psychological problems found in obese children but never used analytic jargon to explain anything. Although we knew she had psychiatric training, we thought of her as a pediatrician like the rest of the senior staff.

I have to assume that during that era, psychoanalysis was thought of as a body of ideas to be kept quite separate from other branches of medicine, or that the particular institutions where I was trained did not consider analytic concepts worthy of much consideration in their medical, pediatric, or psychiatric teaching programs. Certainly in the mid-1940s, at the prestigious Babies Hospital in New York, interns were not systematically exposed to Freud's ideas on child development or psychopathology, even though the hospital did have an effective child psychiatry department where such ideas must have been at least known to the director. I was never assigned to that department during my training there and do not know what school of thought prevailed, but it is my impression, based on brief conversations with the director in later years, that he was, in fact, somewhat hostile to psychoanalysis. This may account for the exclusion of its concepts from our pediatric education.

In spite of all that, I am now a psychoanalyst, and have been one for many years. I graduated from an institute accredited by the American Psychoanalytic Association, remain a member of a rather conservative "classical" local society, and am eligible to join the American as an individual member. When I consider it the treatment of choice, I practice a method of psychoanalysis which I believe to be compatible with the standards of that organization, although in my opinion, for most of my patients, some form of psychotherapy rather than psycho-analysis is the most appropriate form of treatment.

I was attracted to the profession primarily by the fact that even before I knew much about psychoanalysis, life experience had convinced me of the power that unconscious motivation exerted over my own behavior. Awareness of such forces within myself was reinforced dramatically by seeing them in action on a children's psychiatric service, and I felt a strong need to know more about how the mind works. I needed to know not only through personal experience in my own analysis but through the kind of detailed observation of mental processes that can be attained only by analyzing others. Interest in Freud and his theories came after I was already involved, not the other way around, as is so often the case with analysts I have known.

A lot of what Freud said about child development made sense to me, and still does, even though research in other fields has added much to his original formulations and cast doubt on some of his original ideas. I had spent considerable time observing the behavior of infants and small children, both as a pediatrician and as consultant in a number of nursery schools over a protracted period of time, and my own observations seemed to confirm much of what Freud had reconstructed from the analyses of adults.

Just to take one instance, anyone who has heard over and over again the outraged "where is mine?" response of little girls to the first sight of a little boy's penis cannot doubt that at least at the age of two or three penis envy is alive and well. This concept is a major target of feminist groups in their attacks on psychoanalysis, and it has obviously suffered by the tendency to denigrate women's anger at all the inequities they encounter later in life through reducing the cause of that anger to early childhood wishes for a penis. I resent these realistic injustices as much as any woman does. However, to discard altogether the idea that early penis envy existed is just as unrealistic as to blame it for everything women later feel toward men. The same goes for a lot of other things that Freud hypothesized.

I am not a theoretician and do not want to be. My primary interest has always been therapeutic. But I am also dedicated to obtaining data in support of theories proposed by others, and in support of the interpretations I make in my clinical work. "Where is your evidence, Dr. Parker?" I can still hear the clear, cool voice of Dr. Alexander at Babies Hospital, and that of Miss Littell at the Brearley School. "Make your own observations and then see how they fit with what others have said." That is what has interested me. It is what I try to do in working with my patients, and the purpose of everything I have written is to furnish concrete material for others to use in the same way if they wish.

I have spent a great deal of time and money in becoming an analyst and have great respect for "classical" psychoanalysis, both as a clinical and as a theoretical system. I am grateful for the training, which I feel imposed a valuable discipline on my clinical work, not only that which is strictly psychoanalysis as defined by my colleagues, but also that defined as psychotherapy. I am proud to belong to a group of people most of whom I consider sincere, scholarly seekers after truth as they see it, and believe I have a pretty good professional reputation among them. However, I do not consider myself a "member of the establishment" and take no part in professional politics, which are complicated and often strident. I am not an "organization woman."

Speculation about fine points of theory at high levels of abstraction does not interest me, nor do arguments about whether an analyst who proposes changes in theory or technique has forfeited the right to be called an analyst. These are the kinds of discussions that seem to interest many of my colleagues at society meetings that I have attended, and I don't attend as many meetings as I might for that reason. I would be very much interested in hearing good discussions of clinical case material and the details of interactions between analyst and patient, but these seldom occur, and I find this disappointing. A senior colleague once said to me rather plaintively, "You do good work, but you don't think like an analyst." From his point of view, he was perfectly right. I don't think the way he does, or the way a lot of my colleagues do. I respect their points of view, and I can also understand why mine sometimes differs.

I never had the privilege of being in at the birth of a new intellectual movement that in many ways changed ways of thinking throughout at least the Western world. I do not believe in treating Freud's every word as a treasure rescued from a culture on the brink of destruction. Literal adherence to concepts conceived nearly a century ago is not a religion to me as it is to many of my European colleagues and those indoctrinated by them. Their feelings come from a different place than mine.

Along with a good many other reputable, classically trained psychoanalysts, I no longer believe all of Freud's "metapsychology." I also question the way many of his modern followers interpret some of what he said about clinical technique and the nature of the psychoanalytic process. Here, in brief, and greatly simplified, is what I do believe about psychoanalysis.

I believe that psychoanalysis is a process that takes place on the basis of a relationship between two people who interact in a unique way with the goal of promoting deep-seated characterological changes in one of them, the patient. I believe that such changes become possible as the patient gradually develops trust and confidence in the analyst to the point where he or she can relinquish defenses against revealing conscious and unconscious attitudes and feelings which have impeded his or her ability to function adequately.

This is a process that takes place between two real people, not one person and a blank screen, a term by which Freud described what he felt the analyst should be, although in his own work with patients he was anything but a blank screen. Some of his followers have taken this literally and try to remain completely anonymous. I consider this neither desirable nor possible.

No matter how neutral his attitude toward what the patient says (and I believe the analyst should be as neutral as possible), the analyst inevitably reveals a good deal about himself or herself. I know of one who tried to reduce all environmental stimuli in his office by draping the walls with black curtains. Can you imagine anything more revealing about that analyst? Inevitably, the way he or she dresses and furnishes the office—the tones of voice, the kinds of statements by the patient commented upon or not commented upon—all such things and many others, including things gleaned by the patient from outside sources, give the patient many clues to the personality of the analyst. In my opinion, it is not so much what the patient knows about the analyst or what happens in the transaction between them that is important. What is important is whether the patient's feelings and interpretations of such matters get discussed and understood, not only in terms of the transference but often also in terms of realities in the here and now.

I do not believe that changes in the patient take place purely as a result of correct interpretations by the analyst. I believe that the trust necessary to bring about change develops on the basis of a relationship with the analyst, some of which is based on transference and some of which is based on what actually happens between them—the degree to which the patient perceives the analyst as honest, reasonable, and dedicated to the success of their work.

Often a patient perceives the analyst in a way that has been distorted by his past experience, but not always. Sometimes his perceptions are perfectly correct and relevant to what he is feeling about the analyst at the moment, and sometimes it is appropriate for the analyst to confirm this, removing from the patient the onus of losing faith in his own perceptions. Sometimes it is appropriate for the analyst to answer a reasonable question as well as to analyze why the question was asked. Sometimes it is also appropriate for the analyst to question why the patient is obeying all the rules of the analysis as well as to raise questions when the patient is not. I know of a patient who, when temporarily drained of funds by a family emergency, went out and borrowed money at high interest in order to avoid delaying payment to the analyst for a week. The analyst never questioned what to my mind was quite irrational behavior on the patient's part.

These are the kinds of things in which I differ from the strictly classical ideas on technique, and I am glad to say that many of my classically trained colleagues agree completely.

In such matters I differ from those who may still be a majority in the profession, but I can respect their point of view. What I cannot respect, however, is the arrogance with which those people assume that anyone who fails to accept all their views on theory or technique has lost the right to be called a psychoanalyst.

This latter point has been a hot political issue since the beginning of the psychoanalytic movement and has led to many of the splits and animosities that plague the profession. It has caused many of the most creative thinkers, both those in the early days and more recently, to break from the mainstream of analysis and has stifled the free flow of ideas within professional societies still within the mainstream.

A scientific atmosphere is one where traditional concepts can be challenged and controversial ideas introduced without invoking fear that anyone who disagrees with prevailing views will no longer be considered an acceptable member of the profession by his or her colleagues. Psychoanalysts consider themselves scientists, but this kind of atmosphere does not exist in many analytic societies today any more than it did in the days of Freud. Quite the conrary, in fact. In order to challenge traditional views, groups of people originally united by their interest in Freud's ideas have had to break away from mainstream psychoanalysis, and those who still adhere to the strictly classical position actually fear having their candidates exposed to the ideas of those who are now considered deviant. Thus various streams of analytic thought have grown up in isolation from each other, and each has developed a literature of its own which is not only unread by those in other streams of thought but is often actually prohibited.

I can illustrate the above by two occasions described to me by an analyst with eclectic interests in the field—one who is internationally esteemed as a teacher and lecturer. After lecturing to a group of orthodox analytic candidates in the Middle West, he was asked by one of them for references about an idea in the lecture which had interested the student. When given the reference, the candidate (a man in his middle forties, by the way) replied sadly, "I'm sorry, but candidates in our Institute are not allowed to read Sullivan." This same teacher and lecturer, invited by the education committee of another orthodox institute to address candidates, was warned that only the fourth-year students would be allowed to come, for fear that the lecturer would "seduce" the others with unorthodox ideas. (Presumably by the fourth year, students are sufficiently indoctrinated so as to be impervious to deviant thoughts.) To me, this kind of training is not only unscientific but very sad.

I have been fortunate. My husband, Otto Will, was trained in an orthodox institute back in the days when Harry Stack Sullivan and Frieda Fromm-Reichman were still on the faculty. Sullivan, an American psychiatrist, was among those who first became interested in Freud's ideas when they began to become known in this country. He was influential in the early organizations of American analysts and as a matter of fact, was once a-vice-president of the American Psychoanalytic Association. However, he came to believe that Freud had underestimated the role of interpersonal relationships in human development and evolved some theoretical ideas which influenced a great many people, particularly those concerned with trying to understand schizophrenia. He became anathema to mainstream classical analysts, and to the best of my knowledge nowadays no analytic training program that has a course in comparative analytic theories including a study of Sullivan's works is accredited by the American Psychoanalytic Society.

Although Otto became a training analyst in the Washington Psychoanalytic Institute and a member of the American, he was analyzed by both Frieda Fromm-Reichman and Sullivan, who greatly influenced him. Since our marriage, he has exposed me to some of the so-called interpersonal theories and literature. Those who espouse these ideas are not considered real analysts by the more classical groups, but I have found that talking with Otto about clinical matters has widened my own professional horizon enormously and has not "contaminated" me to the point where I am considered less of a real analyst by my colleagues.

In journals that I never heard of before, I have read articles that are totally relevant and not at all in conflict with the way I think about my work. The ways in which Otto and I look at our profession are complementary, not antagonistic, and I believe that our sharing of differences in training and experience has enriched us both. Fortunately we consider each other to be real analysts who, in spite of some differences in emphasis, believe in all the elements of psychoanalytic theory that are basic to the field and are shared by analysts of both classical and interpersonal orientation. I wish I could see this kind of open-minded sharing of sometimes controversial ideas at meetings of my professional society, but the day when that can occur has not yet arrived.

Some kind of official definition of a psychoanalyst may become a necessity in the future, when third-party health care payers become incresingly influential in determining legitimate forms of treatment. I do not believe that the classical analysts will be able to lay sole claim to the use of this title and can only hope that the title will not become meaningless through widespread use by insufficiently trained analytic groups which are at present proliferating at an alarming rate.

It is my hope that eventually, to legitimize the title for qualified analysts, an organization will be formed which includes the graduates of all reputable psychoanalyltic training schools that offer rigorous programs in the basics of analytic belief that are shared by all. Such programs include intensive study of Freud's work along with whatever other theories are considered and offer their candidates intensive supervision in the conduct of a least three clinical cases regardless of differences in the kinds of technique taught. Although they differ on points of emphasis, well-trained analysts with both a classical and an interpersonal orientation have a great deal in common, and much to lose by ignoring each other's ideas. If such an organization is formed within my lifetime, I shall be motivated to participate wholeheartedly, but I am not holding my breath waiting for it to happen.

On Tolerating Uncertainty

Now I am seventy-five years old. I guess the last chapter of life is beginning, although it could be a long one. Never forget those genes! Both my parents and all but one of my grandparents lived into their late eighties, and a paternal aunt died only recently at the age of ninety-eight. Never, however, discount the power of factors in the environment which may alter the influence of genetic potential, both for good and for bad.

Beautiful San Francisco Bay, where I used to swim just off the front of my garden, is now polluted by deadly PCBs. The Standard Oil refinery, less than a mile away, still exudes noxious fumes now and then, despite improvements in filtration since the day in the 1940s when a chemical mist, blown our way by the north wind, took the paint off our house. Who knows what such things have done to reduce the natural resistances to deterioration of which our bodies are capable? This is not to speak of nuclear missiles planted all over the world which could blow everyone up before the end of the century. Who knows whether the human race can survive man's ever-increasing ingenuity?

In order to avoid recognizing their fears of their own imminent demise, older people sometimes tend to dwell on dangers in the surrounding environment or to deny them and develop an undesirable sense of complacency. I don't wish to do either of those things, but it is sometimes difficult to strike a reasonable balance between them.

The world has always been filled with physical hazards and threats to the psychological stability of people who can be traumatized by rapid changes in their society. Such changes have taken place at an accelerating pace throughout the generations, particularly in the United States, where life changed from struggle against the wilderness to struggle against the complexities of a highly industrialized nation within relatively few generations. Think of the adjustments required of people in the generation of my grandparents, who were born close to the beginning of Queen Victoria's reign and didn't die until just before we entered World War II. They lived through the revolution caused by the use of electricity and the onset of the automobile and airplane age, saw the structure of societies all over the world toppled by World War I, saw the development of movies, then talking movies and radio. I'm sure many of them were as shocked by the flappers who smoked and drank hard liquor as many people of my age are shocked by drug use and free sexuality among young people to day—sometimes including their own children.

I cannot say that the changes taking place today are having a more drastic effect on my life than those changes had on theirs, but in some ways, recent technological changes have created a situation new to history. Nuclear power has for the first time given man the power to destroy not only himself but most of the life on this planet, animal and vegetable. None of the generations before us had to cope with such an awesome possibility.

Television and computers have now put people all over the world in touch with one another as never before, but at the same time have showed them how far apart they are in their ways of thinking. Nobody who watches the nightly news can escape wondering how these differences can be resolved before someone precipitates a catastrophe.

I should like to think that all people, young or old, are thinking about what steps, however small, they can take to help our world leaders avoid the path to destruction and that they will take these steps, whatever they may be. I feel myself to be in the category of those whose possibilities for action are limited to talking, writing letters and supporting individuals and organizations who have more power to shape events directly. The temptation to despair is never entirely eliminated, but I try to involve myself with various interests closer to home to keep me from brooding about what might happen to the world and from destroying what capacity I may have to be useful & enjoy the rest of my life.

As a matter of fact, I look forward with a certain eagerness to seeing what happens next—what further changes will take place during my lifetime to alter the world I have known. Perhaps, after all, I did get enough milk and TLC in my infancy to ensure that along with a certain basic skepticism, I managed to develop a reasonable basic trust.

My mother used to say "You know you are getting old when policemen begin to look like boys." If that is so, I've been old for a long time, but I refuse to believe it. I'm often surprised when I realize that other people look upon me as old. I feel more as my grandmother did when, on her eighty-ninth birthday, I teasingly said, "I'll bet you feel as young as you did when you were twenty." "No," she replied firmly, "I do not. But I do feel as young as I did when I was sixty." That's about where it's at for me.

So far, old age doesn't seem as bad as it's cracked up to be. So long as I have all my teeth and most of my hair—so long as my mental faculties are still more or less intact and my joints only creak a little—there is a lot left in life to keep me feeling relatively young and spry. Sometimes I be come aware of how many years have gone by only when I notice how many things have changed in my lifetime, but changes seem to take place so fast these days that even they are poor indicators of time's passage. In many ways the changes themselves are a source of interest which keeps me feeling young.

One of the things that interest me is coming to know the children and grandchildren of my friends and neighbors who are now adult—seeing how things have come out for them and speculating about what they will do with their lives in the future. As a avid reader of detective stories, I like to note whether I picked up the proper clues to predict what kinds of people they would become—who managed to succeed in spite of early handicaps, and who managed to lose out after early successes. I also get a certain amount of fun from seeing how some things change in the fashions and then come around full circle to where they were when I was young.

At this stage of the game, I keep thinking back to conversations with my mother when she was where I am now. I can remember being amazed that she seemed to be up on quite a lot of the popular tunes, and a little disgruntled to learn that many of them were merely adaptations of the ones to which she herself danced in her early days. Now I am in the same position; hardly a day goes by that I don't hear a tune from the twenties on my car radio. The same goes for other things too.

Not long ago a young woman came to see me with stars in her eyes saying, "I just found the most wonderful things in a funky old clothes store! Satin nightgowns!" If she had spent as many hours as I have spent in ironing satin nightgowns she would be thanking God for nylon, but it was interesting to hear that the past isn't as completely past as it might sometimes seem. Right now, the dress fashion styles of the twenties are back, while other aspects of the twenties and thirties have never gone away. Clark Gable and Gary Cooper on the TV screen have remained as young and romantic throughout the years as they first looked to us at the neighborhood movie theater. At moments it might seem that sixty years have not gone by at all, but they have. Some things will never be the same again.

Since I grew up and entered upon a career, lots of attitudes have changed in the United States. There is still a long way to go before social justice will be achieved, but little by little, progress is being made in a number of areas. There are still many inequalities between men and women, but in this country it is now no longer strictly a man's world, and women today are considered not only to have the right to enter what were hitherto thought of as men's professions, but in many cases it is assumed that they will do so if they are at all able. Opportunities that I obtained only by the good luck of being in exactly the right place at the right moment in history are now quite generally available to women, in spite of greatly increased competition with men and with other women for acceptance at the most prestigious training facilities. Except for the enormous cost of education and training, there is nothing to stop them from going wherever they want to go.

In my generation, it often took either a world crisis, war, and depression, or personal crisis such as occurred in my family to force people from reasonably comfortable homes into a way of life much different from that of their parents. That is no longer so, and it seems to me that the nature of present-day society is such that probably few young people can grow up without knowing that not only their physical environment but their expectations, opportunities, and value systems may undergo dramatic changes several times in the course of their lives. The children of parents in my generation have already experienced emotional fall-out from the atomic bomb and the anxieties it has created; many have come to doubt the future of life itself.

Fantastic technological advances have already created great potential for changes in our way of life. These can be both good and bad, sometimes both at the same time. Take as one small example what has recently happened in medicine.

For generations before my time, methods of diagnosis and treatment were relatively primitive. Infection was a major cause of death, and its treatment consisted largely of prescribing rest, liquids, and a fervent hope that the body's own recuperative forces would be strong enough to overpower the germs. Then came the discovery of specific sera to increase immunity to various kinds of bacteria, but not until as late as just before my own years of internship and residency in the early 1940s did doctors begin to have the use of specific drugs like sulfadiazine and penicillin to deal with a wide range of infectious agents.

In the last forty years there has been a virtual revolution not only in the drug industry but in the whole diagnostic and therapeutic armamentarium through the development of machinery such as the electron microscope and C.A.T. scanners. I have no doubt at all that these will soon be outdated and replaced by even more effective tools, and that these will further change the practice of medicine probably even faster than did those we use now. All these advances have been of great benefit to both patients and doctors, but for doctors they have also created problems which are very likely to affect the way they practice their profession.

When Alberta and I first came west after our training at Babies Hospsital, she was starting a pediatric practice and one night received an emergency call through the answering service to see a critically ill baby in a housing project.

It was not until after she had already examined the child, and was about to start treatment, that she discovered the whole family was under the care of an aging general practitioner in the area. In calling him to explain how she happened to be on the case, she described her findings and asked whether he wanted to take over or whether she should carry on with her proposed treatment. He replied, "Oh, by all means take over the case, and do whatever you want. The babies with that condition always die anyway, of course."

Well, that particular baby didn't have to die anyway. It had an infectious disease which had indeed been fatal until a few years previously, but was by then readily treatable with sulfadiazine, a drug that was still quite new but familiar to any recently trained doctor. That general practitioner might not have been one of the brightest and the best, but I suspect he was not alone among doctors of his generation in ignorance of the latest discoveries, and I'm reasonably sure that there is more than one doctor in that position today when new drugs for all kinds of conditions come out almost daily. I know it is true in psychiatry, and it has put a burden on those practitioners who want to stay up to date. Widespread use of new medical technology has created something of a crisis for doctors in a number of other ways as well. For one thing, raised expectations of miraculous results from wonder drugs and miracle machines, in an increasingly litigious society, has resulted in the need for astronomical amounts of malpractice insurance coverage, and the huge cost of premiums is literally threatening to drive many doctors out of high-risk specialties. Only recently I listened to a TV documentary on how certain small towns in New York State may lose all their orthopedists, obstetricians, and radiologists because the price of insurance has become intolerable, and no doubt the same kind of thing will soon be happening in other states. Even practitioners in the supposedly low-risk specialties, such as analysts and psychotherapists like my self who do not use electric shock or psychotropic drugs are not immune to the possibility of being sued. Even though there is considerable controversy among reputable psychiatrists about the advisability of using such things in particular kinds of cases, it is quite conceivable that if the results of treatment seem unsatisfactory, one might be sued for not using them. This kind of situation is a source of considerable frustration.

Since both hospitals and doctors have had to increase fees to cover direct and indirect costs of medical technology, costs to patients of medical care have risen to a point where introduction of third-party payers has become necessary to share the burden—insurance companies and government agencies. These agencies, in an attempt to make medical care cost-effective, are moving into the position of becoming standard setters for the forms of treatment that doctors may employ.

Emphasis on cost-effectiveness is in the process of changing the whole system of health care delivery, and may eventually bring about elimination of the solo practitioner almost completely.

Gone will be the kind of doctor who maintained long-term ongoing relationships with patients and determined their care solely on the basis of what he or she considered to be their needs. Gone, also, will be a major source of satisfaction that many doctors have derived from practicing medicine. Medicine is a profession involving heavy responsibility and considerable physical as well as emotional strain. When a close knowledge of patients as people, and pleasure in human relationships between doctor and patient, can no longer be depended upon to offset the frustrations and stresses, the attitudes of many toward their work may change a good deal. When doctors are no longer free to use their own judgment and are under increasing control over the way they work—when the practice of medicine ceases to be an art and becomes more and more just a business to make money, what will happen to the profession? Will women who are now entering medical schools in considerable numbers want to choose the field if these kinds of satisfactions are no longer to be derived from it? Will the same kinds of caring young people who, for the most part were those who chose to go into medicine in the past continue to do so? Right now, medicine is a profession of great prestige, particularly among women who have hitherto been largely excluded from the higher-paying occupations and are eager to take their place in the sun. Nurturant and interpersonal aspects of the work have been among the biggest attractions. Will those already in it want to stay?

I have already talked to several young doctors who openly admit that they plan to practice only long enough to gain financial security. I have already seen among my acquaintances a number of older doctors leave medicine at the height of their careers to enter business, or buy vineyards because they think they see the kind of practice that has been satisfying to them disappearing. A number of psychiatrists who entered the field out of an interest in working with people are leaving it with the feeling that the profession will soon be reduced to pill-pushing. These are all people who thought their careers were assured, but have found that social changes imposed on their field by modern technology require of them an entirely new orientation.

Are there today any kinds of jobs for which the young can prepare with absolute assurance that the job will not become obsolete, or that its requirements and the satisfactions to be derived from it will not have been altered after a while? Is there any kind of professional training that may not be at least partially outmoded before the trainee is well launched on his or her career? Are there any values or social mores that may not be reversed at least once within every generation?

These are questions for which I have no answers. However, I believe that those who can tolerate not having them answered will be the ones best fitted to meet challenges in an increasingly complicated world. They will be the people who have been brought up from the start to tolerate uncertainty and change, and to meet unexpected events, including personal setbacks, without being incapacitated by anxiety.

In many ways my own upbringing was anything but ideal. But as I review my life it seems to me that in regard to being a survivor, I was well trained, whether my parents thought about it that way or not. Partly due to my father's philosophy in regard to raising children and partly to the preoccupation of everyone in the family with his business troubles during my grade-school years, I was encouraged, indeed almost forced to develop the independence and initiative to cope with my own problems that is the cornerstone of survivorship. This was reinforced later by the changes and uncertainties met in adolescence and early adult life which made it necessary to develop tolerance for an almost constant sense of insecurity.

In spite of all the ambivalences and conflicts of loyalty in early childhood, I obviously got enough feeling of being loved, protected, and respected for my accomplishments to reach school age with the ability to leaarn and gain skills. From that time on, although I had plenty of supervision and discipline, I was essentially trusted to take care of my own affairs and get out of trouble by my own intiative.

On the first day of school I was told that just as my Daddy's job was to earn money, and Mother's job to run the household, my job was to do my schoolwork and get along with my teachers and new friends. From then on, I was left alone to do just that. Nobody urged me to do my homework or helped me get it done. If it wasn't in on time, that was between me and the teacher, and although my mother frequently conferred with my teachers, nobody from home interfered with my life at school. It was simply assumed that I would do my best. I did, and got good grades in everything except "Conduct." That was usually a "C," but whatever discipline was required took place at school and nobody mentioned it at home.

From the age of nine, I lived within bicycling distance of the school and transported myself unless the weather was too bad. My father believed, and I believe to this day, that many upper-middle-class children are overprotected and retarded in developing a sense of independence. "Accidents can happen anywhere," he said, "but if you are careful, they probably won't." I was, and they didn't. I doubt that in the unsafe cities of today such a laissez-faire attitude would be feasible, but at that time, in the part of Chicago where we lived, it was considered quite safe, and I believe the freedom had a salutary effect on me. I valued the trust my parents placed in my good judgment, and did my best to live up to it.

The constant changes that I had to absorb from preadolescence well into adult life were in many ways painful, but they did me an invaluable service by forcing me to adapt not only to a frequently changing environment, but to the differing ideas of a wide range of people, and to do so without letting anxiety overwhelm me. It seems to me that in the uncertain world of today, everyone who is going to survive will have to develop that capacity to some degree.

I believe that in adolescence and early adulthood too great a sense of safety may be a mixed blessing. It may, and quite often does, defer an important step in the development of true, lasting self-confidence which can only be acquired after a young person has faced challenges and learned that he or she has the inner resources to master them.

The amount of anxiety aroused by unexpected hardship in someone who has never had to face any adversity may seem overwhelming. I am sure we have all seen an example of the early-blooming boys and girls who were stars in grade school but faded away at high school and college level where they met real competition and unexpected setbacks. Young people who have never known anything but admiration, praise, and help in everything they attempted may not be as adequately prepared for the real world as those who were allowed to make disappointing choices and recover from them by their own ingenuity. They have not been taught to tolerate the anxieties aroused by meeting the unexpected with assurance.

At an early age, I learned that nothing can be counted on to remain the same, but along with that, I learned that change does not always spell disaster, even when your highest hopes are dashed. Life experience taught me that if you are in a bad situation, you can always retool and move into something different, even though you may lose time and have no assurance that the next thing will be much better. I learned that experience itself is an asset, even if at the time it seemed like a bad one. The ability to put one kind of experience behind me and move into something new without being overwhelmed by anxiety was, I think, an essential element in my development.

Although I hate to admit it, I attribute some of this ability to bombardment from my parents with maxims and catchwords. This nearly drove me crazy, but I am still surprised today at how many of them came to mind and goaded me to action in times of stress. "Chalk it up to experience," my mother would say when something went wrong—not unsympathetically, but with a certain wistful fatalism. "Don't send good money after bad" was my father's version of the idea that if you have made an investment of time and energy in something that didn't work out, take your losses and cut loose. To me that was a very valuable idea—the idea that you don't have to stick with something just because you have already put a lot into it.

The assurance that mistakes in judgment are not a disgrace has stayed with me throughout my life, and I have found it useful to many people with whom I have worked professionally. To my mind, the "Right to be wrong" stands right up there with the "Right to life, liberty and the pursuit of happiness," It is very comforting to believe that one can learn from one's mistakes without having to be guilty for having made them. If the story of my life has done nothing else, I hope it has made that point, and shown that uncertainty and the necessity to accept change may lead not only to anxiety but to growth.

So I will end the story by adding to the statement I made in the beginning. Parents can give their children great gifts—gifts which vary according to different stages of their children's lives. They can give children in earliest life the security of feeling loved, protected and respected for their achievements; at school age they can give trust and encouragement to develop confidence in, and responsibility for their own judgment. Past early adolescence, the greatest gift that can be given to young people is freedom to make their own choices, even bad choices, and to rally from mistakes in their own way.

Those gifts were given to me, and I think they got me through.